Grace
in
HORROR

*May the Loving Father
bless you abundantly!*

Fr. Modestus, op

Modestus Ngwu, O.P.

ISBN 978-1-0980-5783-1 (paperback)
ISBN 978-1-0980-5784-8 (hardcover)
ISBN 978-1-0980-5785-5 (digital)

Christian Faith Publishing, Inc.
832 Park Avenue
Meadville, PA 16335
www.christianfaithpublishing.com

While the experiences narrated in this book are true, they constitute the compilation of hundreds of hours of chaplaincy work carried out at the hospital. All names, characters, events, incidents, and personal identifiable information have been disguised and/or changed in order to protect the privacy of the parties involved. Any resemblance to actual persons, living or dead, or actual events is purely coincidental.

Printed in the United States of America

To patients and families to whom I had the privilege
of ministering while standing at their bedside.
You taught me the deeper meaning of grace with your tears and smiles.

The silence of our loving God, in the face of human suffering, perplexes everyone who has ever struggled with this mystery. But when you are a priest and are meant to be the face of the loving God, for others, what do you say, how can you help? Recounting his everyday experiences as a hospital chaplain, Dominican Father, Modestus Ngwu, describes with disarming sincerity and candor his wrestling match with himself, human suffering, and God. When the academic answers and the everyday polite comments failed to console and, sometimes, hurt, he allowed his own raw encounters with patients to teach him a genuine ministry of compassion, to listen, to be present, and to accompany those facing their undeniable vulnerability. Father Modestus' book reveals how grace is truly present and active in what might appear to be utter horror.

Most Rev. Ronald W. Gainer
Bishop of Harrisburg

"There is a magnificent glory hidden and being revealed in suffering."

"Silence creates the space where grace and beauty meet to give birth to love."

These are just two examples of the riches to be found in *Grace in Horror*, a movingly humble and ultimately hopeful reflection written by a hospital chaplain, Fr. Modestus Ngwu, O.P. It chronicles his spiritual journey as a priest encountering horrific suffering among his patients. He asks the honest questions, we all think and fear, about suffering, pain, and death, and the true nature of grace and compassion. He examines through his role as a priest who grieves with his patients the stages of denial, silence, acceptance, redemption, and even rejoicing, and how a person of faith can encounter the God who journeys with us. Fr. Modestus shows how through that pain, the silence, and the questions we can adapt a proper ordered view of the value of suffering and grace. This reflection is highly recommended for anyone in health care, for anyone who asks, *why does a good God allow suffering* and for anyone who seeks to delve deeper into the mysteries of Grace. It is a compelling read that offers much to reflect and meditate upon.

Elizabeth E. Frauenhoffer, MD, OCDS
Professor of Pathology and Orthopaedics
Penn State Health MS Hershey Medical Center
Penn State University College of Medicine
Secretary, Harrisburg Diocesan Guild of the
Catholic Medical Association

Wow, this is an excellent book. I have to admit that I have found it professionally challenging to read at times as much of the context strike very close to home. It has brought me to tears many times as so many of the stories and questions are what I have experience in my life as a physician. It has also brought me much joy as it reaffirmed my role as a physician who's vocation it is to walk with my patients in their horror. It helps me to find solace in knowing that it is only God that gives me and my patients the grace to not only endure but move people from the horror though a journey to grace.

This book for me strips away the fluff of modern niceties and forces one to ask the questions of meaning and substance, just like the psalmists. Suffering is at the heart of human existence, and although it is expected, horror describes concisely what this human experience is. In the modern world, we experience it most dramatically in our institutions of care. This book strikes at the heart of this vexing issue and in a world with so much suffering reaffirms that it is only God that can help us comprehend and endure the difficulties of our lives. These experiences defining not just who we are but who we become. We in healthcare, doctors, nurses, caregivers, and our priest need always remember that we are God tools that help move patients and our colleagues from great Horror back to Gods grace.

I don't know how such a joyful priest can remain joyful in the continuous horror experienced as a hospital chaplain, but I do know this joy is the fruit of something only God can provide.

Mark Bosch, MD. FRCPC. (Internal Medicine & Hematology)
Bone Marrow Transplant Hematologist, Saskatchewan Cancer Agency
Associate Professor, University of Saskatchewan,
Division of Oncology, Sk. Canada

Fr. Modestus has put into words the meaning and experience of lament. Through his tears, he has looked for the divine and found silence. Silence, he says, echoes love. He has taken his personal account as a witness of persons in crisis and communicated that the truth of depth is indeed the appearance of two or more contradictions that are mutually coexisting without one cancelling out the other. Such is the glimpse Modestus has given the reader into the life and work of a priest and chaplain serving in a hospital. In his pages, he has delivered us to the triumph of living a life that embraces tragedy. He shows us the strength of the human spirit woven by the fabric of no longer seeking to overcome life's suffering; rather, he instructs the lament as a pastoral act which allows the person providing care to hear the cry of the sufferer and commune never allowing the person to feel alone. This is a must read for anyone who works in health care and for anyone who asks, "where is God in our suffering.

David Carnish, MA, M/Div. BCC, ACPE Certified Educator
Penn State Hershey Medical Center

This book is fascinating and challenging as it deals with some very difficult issues in an easy to understand manner. We particularly enjoyed and appreciate the references Fr. Modestus made to his childhood in Nigeria and the mesmerizing stories he articulated so well in this book *Grace in Horror*. Those experiences obviously had great influence on his approach to dealing with hospital patients. Working so closely with a great number of seriously ill patients must be exhausting, but he handles those difficult duties with true grace. We believe that this book could very well serve as a text for study and discussion by people involved with counseling patients in hospital settings and those asking to understand 'Why?'

Kit and Bernie Ryan

Acknowledgments

Grace in Horror is a labor of love that would never have been possible without the support, love, hard work, and encouragement of some very special people. Jane Oskutis was the first to recognize that my experiences and struggles as a hospital chaplain had intrinsic value and were worthy of a book that could become a source of comfort to others. There are no words to express my gratitude for her support and belief in me, and for bringing along Virginia Robertson to assist with the compilation and editing of the original manuscript. Countless hours were spent to ensure that a collection of heartfelt thoughts stemming from real-life stories could become a ray of hope to those facing unimaginable brokenness. My eternal and heartfelt gratitude to these two ladies who, each in their own way, were instrumental in the creation of this book. I am eternally grateful to their husbands, Roy Oskutis and Gavin Robertson, who supported and sacrificed their family time with them during the creative process. I also want to thank Rev. Fr. Ignatius Madumere, O.P. for his theological feedback and Kathleen Shovlin for reading an earlier manuscript.

Last but not least, I would like to thank my family and friends. I could not have done this without your love and prayers. Above all, I thank God who made this book possible through His grace.

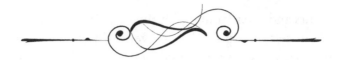

Introduction

Growing up in Nigeria shaped me in ways that I never imagined would help me with my vocation. I have been a Roman Catholic priest for fifteen years. I have embraced and welcomed every aspect of my calling. I have studied, prepared, and looked forward to serving for as long as I can remember. However, my very first experience with hospital chaplaincy took place in 2013 when I was asked to volunteer for two weeks at Saskatoon Hospital. This experience was, in no small sense, a living nightmare. It affected me for weeks.

When I was later approached and asked, "Would you like to do chaplaincy work at the hospital again?" my response did not involve any thinking whatsoever. I remember hearing myself viscerally and categorically saying, "No, thank you!"

At the conclusion of that very emotional initial experience, I had a sensational sense of relief handing the pager back to the chaplain I had been replacing. I was absolutely certain and quite determined to never doing hospital chaplaincy again. Administering six Last Rites within a two-week period had taken a toll on me. Last Rite is a prayer and the ministrations given by a Catholic priest to a patient of the faith who is actively dying. There is no doubt that one of the things that affected me most was ministering to a terminally ill fourteen-month-old boy. I just couldn't bear his family's anguish, his agony, and the overall pain I was witnessing.

Another contributing factor to my reluctance to engaging in chaplaincy work was a sheer inability to schedule my time. I never knew what was going to happen next. The chaplain's phone can ring anytime of the day or night. When that happens, the chaplain is expected to rush to the hospital and attend to the sacramental needs of the patients and their families. During my first volunteering experience, this uncertainty proved to be very distressing. As a priest, I was trained to say prayers for people and console them in their times of suffering. I was taught to offer hope by assuring the faithful that God is with them. As a chaplain, I had to tend to those who suffer and have little hope of recovering as well as to their family members. That was very difficult.

I soon realized that God had quite the sense of humor and that He had His own plans for me, and those plans include hospital chaplaincy. When I was transferred from Saskatoon, Canada, to Harrisburg PA, USA in 2016, do you know my assignment? Hospital chaplaincy in Hershey Medical Center. The truth is that I dreaded working at the hospital. I have to admit that I was tempted to just pay someone else so long as I didn't have to do it. I was truly hoping that my assignment would only last for six months, at which time I could move on with my life. However, God had His own plans. He placed me in the midst of pain, tears, and the brokenness of the hospital. Being with people in their darkest hours transported me to places beyond my imagination and allowed me to appreciate things I had taken for granted. God, throughout it all, blessed me with His grace. Starting a new ministry at the hospital was a terrifying struggle for me. It was difficult to find grace in hospital ministry, especially having to witness the terrible suffering endured by patients.

This work was inspired by my struggles with brokenness and the grace I found in the most unexpected of places. It is also a narrative of hospital experiences. There, I found horror interspersed with unimaginable grace. It also depicts the cries and lamentations shared by thousands of people around the world who bemoan human powerlessness in the face of suffering. We seek answers, and we yearn to find human responses to circumstances that go beyond our comprehension. We clamor for help, and we seemingly hear silence. We pray, and our prayers are not heard. God seems absent. I will attempt to address these issues and describe what I say to those who are hurting, broken, and crushed by sickness, crisis, and all kinds of astonishing suffering. I will also be discussing the merits and pitfalls of the phrases often used by well-intended people when dealing with illnesses, suffering, and death itself. I will be writing a distress letter to God. It will not be a defiant letter, but I will share the raw brokenness and vulnerability I also experience in the midst of suffering.

Part I

THE LAMENT

"Weeping may last through the night, but joy
comes with the morning" (Psalm 30:5).

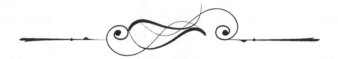

Bemoaning Powerlessness

During the winter of 2017, I was asked to baptize a dying three-month-old baby in the Intensive Care Unit. I saw this very beautiful little girl, adorably dressed. I saw the mom showering love on her daughter. After the baptism, I was asked to stay because she was expected to die soon. I waited while she was being extubated. The baby was gently placed in her mother's arms. I blessed the child while her mother held her, rocking her and singing to her through her tears until the baby took her last breath. I stood there shattered, in shock, bewildered, and crushed as if I was hit by a heavy rock. I wanted to run away from the hospital. I couldn't bear it. I was devastated. After that whole experience, I was not quite sure how I managed to get to my supervisor's office, but I broke down as soon as I arrived. We could speculate and theologize about suffering indefinitely, but being in the midst of suffering feels very different.

That is maybe why we find little solace when we are told, "In everything, give thanks and be positive." We are also often told, "God called her for a reason! He or she is no longer suffering. He or she is in a better place." We are also not strangers to the following assertion, "She is now an angel in heaven." Actually, how many times have we been told to trust God in times of distress and that "everything happens for a reason and for our own good"? Some of us may also have heard the expression, "Offer it up for the souls in purgatory and those who are suffering." I guess it is also safe to assume that we have heard of the term *redemptive suffering*, even though we may not fully understand its theological implication. There have been times when people have invited us to unite our suffering with God's: "God will ease the suffering of thousands of people in the world because we are uniting our suffering with the suffering of Jesus." These well-meaning people have learned or heard these phrases and use them in an attempt to support and comfort us in times of difficulty.

Unfortunately, these responses to grief do not address the deep hurt that we experience. Sometimes they even sound like an attempt to defend God. We are drawn to an institutionalized ideal of a God who has all the answers. We are taught to listen and obey Him. We are told to believe in His will for us and that our own will is secondary to His. We are presented with different theological propositions in times of suffering that appear to defend God. Does God really need us to defend Him in times of suffering? Do we need to continue to offer answers to assign meaning to human suffering? Do we really need to defend God, or should we allow God to be God? Theological answers may be adequate intellectually, but they fail to give our pain, fear, and anxiety any space. They fail to acknowledge our existence and the reality of our hurt. They fail to give meaning to our tears and fears.

Everyone experiences suffering in one way or another, directly or indirectly. It may be physical, social, economic, or psychological suffering. The list of human suffering is endless. The fact that we are oblivious to people's suffering because we see them laugh, play, or act stoic does not mean they are exempt. Being a celebrity, reality TV star, social media influencer, and having all the money in the world does not exempt us. Even when we want to ignore the suffering of others, it stares us right in the face. It is unavoidable as we listen to the news and see our friends and family suffer. Everyone's experience of suffering is different, be it divorce, sickness, financial crisis, poverty, losses, obesity, anorexia, loneliness, and feelings of worthlessness. They all constitute suffering.

It is no secret that many people cannot or do not know how to deal with pain. It is natural to try to avoid it and not want to talk about it or face it. We do our best to shut it down, run away from it, forget it, and not deal with it. However, sickness and pain are an unavoidable reality from which we cannot run away. Therefore, we doubt the benevolence of God, His omnipotence and omnipresence, but dare not say that. We do not want to be labelled as doubters of our faith. The inability to give voice to our suffering causes us to experience powerlessness, loneliness, abandonment, emptiness, and worthlessness. This psychological suffering can be worse than any physical suffering. It pushes us to hopelessness and despair as the experience of alienation increases. So what do we do? We keep our mouths shut. We become silent while our hearts bleed with more unanswered questions, guilt, and hurt. We prefer to remain quiet and live with those doubts than add shame and humiliation to it. We bottle them up. We suffer not only the physical pain but the psychological affliction of not having answers.

Some resort to drugs, alcohol, or other destructive behavior to cope with suffering. A much healthier option would be to remain open to the grace of God in the midst of our suffering. To experience this grace, we must understand grace. What do we mean by grace?

Through my everyday experiences at the hospital, I have learned that grace is not as simple as what we were taught. There is a dazzling mystery in grace as it is revealed to us. The Grace in Horror is transformative and allows us to learn from it, thus restoring us.

Through the biblical account of the story of the Israelites, we see the grandeur of grace. The Israelites learned that God was with them throughout their history, particularly in times of famine, war, disease, and death. We see that God made His caring presence known to them. Grace is what helps us transform our helplessness into something meaningful.

For many patients, being diagnosed with cancer, MS, or any terminal disease is devastating. Their whole world crumbles. When I come upon those who are broken, I allow myself to be broken with them. I share in their pain, suffering, tears, prayers, and hope. I join them in their silence while they wait, search, and hope for the fulfilment of God's promise to us: "Be strong and courageous. Do not be afraid or terrified because of them, for the Lord your God goes with you; he will never leave you nor forsake you" (Deuteronomy 31:6).

In spite of this promise, we falter. My dialect uses the expression "Akwa ariri!" (unending, deep-rooted painful groaning). This is the sort of scream that leaves no tears unshed and causes red eyes and bleeding hearts. It is the type of cry that carries so much pain that it chokes us. When we cry out loud like that, it echoes in the distance.

This hurt is so painful and real that it drives us to dark areas in our soul. When this happens, our reasoning freezes, time freezes, life freezes, and everything around us freezes. We scream, but no words come out. When we want to stand up, we cannot move. At that moment, words seem empty and worthless; what anyone says to us is devoid of relevance and meaning. We are beaten down and lack the words to express the depth of our fears. This way of screaming may not make sense, but no one would wish to be in this state of darkness.

Coming face-to-face with suffering daily at the hospital was frightful for me. It broke my heart and left me speechless. I saw myself asking fundamental questions that I thought I was already trained to face and had answers for. I wanted to run away because I knew in my heart that there was no way I could deal with the emotional struggle. In the face of this terrible suffering and tears, all the theological answers I had prepared just collapsed.

Upon this calamitous and disastrous suffering, we have been superfluously taught to accept powerlessness as the will of God. Instead of vigorously fighting, praying, and asking God for healing, defaulting to the will of God becomes an escape into powerlessness. "Naked I came from my mother, and naked I will return. The Lord has given; the Lord has taken away; blessed be the name of the Lord" (Job 1:21). For centuries, there has been a fascination with submitting to the will of God by referencing Jesus in His examples and teaching. "Father, if you are willing, take this cup from me. Yet not my will but thine be done!" (Luke 22:42). This unintentionally obscures Jesus's ministry on earth both through His life and teaching. Proclaiming His mission, He said, "The Spirit of the Lord is on me, because he has anointed me to proclaim good news to the poor. He has sent me to proclaim freedom for the prisoners and recovery of sight for the blind, to set the oppressed free, to proclaim. The year of the Lord's favor" (Luke 4:18–19). How on earth did we arrive at this understanding that suffering is God's will for His children? How can it be that Jesus came to liberate the oppressed if God, His Father, is the source of the same oppression?

I continued to reflect and ask myself these questions which I thought I shouldn't really be asking. Please don't feel that as a priest, I should understand and trust God in the face of suffering. Don't tell me to have faith in God and that He knows the plans He has for us. God's plan is not clear when we feel He removed the carpet from underneath our feet. I even asked Him to give me a GPS. So hopefully, no matter how far away from the correct road I may be, I can still move toward my destination. I will eventually get there. We are left in the dark and uncertain. I remember what happened to Zachariah, John the Baptist's father, when the angel appeared to him telling him that his wife, Elizabeth, would conceive and bear him a son, and he doubted. He became dumb until John the Baptist was born. As a minister of God, I should know to trust God as He has all the answers. When witnessing horrendous suffering, those answers no longer seem sufficient.

At first, it was easy for me to be strong and priestly while administering the sacraments, especially Last Rites. I was able to do that once, twice, or periodically. To be confronted with suffering over and over again while working at the hospital shredded me. I couldn't make sense of it anymore. It left me with no choice but to raise these questions and ask God *why*? I know that it may sound like the wrong question to ask, but my faith was seeking understanding. I wanted to find answers to really believe and build my own faith in God. Watching as a child died, I could not continue to bring myself to accept that theodicy makes sense. Filled with tears, I have asked, Where are You, God, when Your children are crushed by pain, sickness, and death? What use is praying to You when You seem far from us in times of need? We prayed, believed the testimonies of what You have done for others; why are You not listening to us and healing those we are asking You to help? We can only speculate about His response to these questions. Why is He deaf to our supplications? Is God really using these experiences to test us as He tested Job? Is He allowing us to suffer so we learn from it? I do not know! Do we really have to go through excruciating suffering, abandonment, hurts, diseases, and pandemics to appreciate the beauty in life? Is God making us go through hell? Really? For what purpose?

I can't believe in God because others say so or because this is all I have ever known. In essence, I have had to find meaning and answers for myself. If I was going to be useful to others in their most difficult times at the hospital, I needed to find grace for myself.

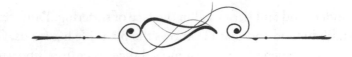

Stunned by Suffering

Visits to the hospital are often unplanned and unexpected. They can cause anxiety and disorientation to patients and loved ones alike. The hospital is a place that really brings out the best and the worst in us all. When hospitalized, we lay down all the power and authority we think we possess. We surrender our freedom, space, and our will to the doctors, nurses, and other hospital staff. They enter our rooms as they deem necessary. "Is it okay if I check your blood pressure?" as if we're really allowed to say no! Our freedom and privacy are gone. We are ready to accept anything provided that we recover and are able to be restored to health. We are open to doing everything possible to feel well again.

Once we are hospitalized, the pain, the fear, and the anxiety looming over us are inescapable. Every human being is afraid of the unknown. We want to have knowledge about the things that are happening around us. We set strategic plans in order to avoid chaos. When we are at the hospital, our plans go out the window. We lie in bed as the body aches, and we are terrified about what we cannot control. We see the bright lights shining in our room, yet our hearts are clouded by darkness.

Many questions begin to loom, and people who had led good Christian lives begin to wonder why God blessed those who ignored Him with good health, a happy family, and wealth while He shuffles those who obey Him from one cross to another? Why is God seemingly disinterested in helping when we need Him? Why didn't God remove the pain and suffering in our lives so we could better serve him? If our help comes from the Lord, why does He not help in times of need? Like the psalmist said, "I lift up my eyes to the mountains—where does my help come from? My help comes from the Lord, the Maker of heaven and earth" (Psalm 121:1).

Could God have prevented cancer, leukemia, MS, and other terrible diseases? Yes! Why did He not? Is He capable of intervening to stop something bad from happening? Yes! Why did He not for a six-year-old boy that I saw in the trauma bay in the emergency department? Being just one minute late could have saved him from the drunk driver who hit him as he rode his bicycle. The accident affected his spinal cord, and he was paralyzed for life.

Where is God when our loved ones suffer from loneliness, addiction, mental illness, drug overdose, or suicide? Where is His love, compassion, abundant grace, and care? We can't see it. Where is our Protector when people we know are shot and killed? A patient once asked me after a long silence, "Why did God allow me to be the only survivor in that car accident? My whole family is gone!" Where is God when a child dies after six months of life? Could God have stopped that? Yes! Why did He not? Could He prevent those things from happening? Yes! Why does He not? Why should we have faith in a God that is distant and not there to help when we suffer? I do not understand God. This silence is why atheists make fun of our faith.

I endeavored to delve deeper into the matter, and my heart cried out to Him as I recalled so many other instances of devastation happening around our world. I asked him, "Why do You watch silently as Your children are in pain? Do You not see your children suffering cancer, leukemia, mental illness, accidents, miscarriages, and being gunned down on the streets? Are You not aware of all the calamities, earthquakes, hurricanes, volcanic eruptions, and other disasters? Why are You not doing anything to stop these atrocities?"

We can go even further by surmising, Does God derive pleasure in seeing us suffer and going through hell so we can prove our faith to Him as Job did? Do our tears make Him happy? Is God sadistic and vengeful? Is He looking at us from heaven and rejoicing in our suffering? How does He express His love for us when we suffer when He is capable and yet fails to help? Why did God punish the rich man in Luke's Gospel (Luke 16:19-31) for not having compassion for Lazarus if He is in heaven celebrating with all the angels and cherubims? They are singing praises in His presence while many families on earth live in pain, suffer, and die horrible deaths. Is he watching Syria, Afghanistan, Iraq, Yemen, South Sudan, and other parts of the world go up in flames?

In times of suffering, it would seem that God does not care. A man stomped out of a church service yelling, "I just can't believe I have all these things to deal with, and you are telling me God loves me, and I should thank Him for giving me this crap? I don't think He cares." Living in pain definitely blurs our belief that God loves us. The pain of perceived abandonment by God is reechoed by the psalmist, "I say to my God my rock, 'Why have you forgotten me? Why must I go about mourning, oppressed by my enemy?' My bones suffer mortal agony as my foes taunt me, saying to me all day long, 'Where is your God?'" (Psalm 42:10).

Jesus, in His life, epitomized this feeling of loneliness and abandonment in his experience at Gethsemane (Luke 22:39–46). With the awareness of the agony He was to undergo, He prayed to God to remove the cross from Him. God was invariably silent to Jesus's plea in the same manner as we feel His silence when we ask for healing at the hospital. The support that Jesus incarnate was hoping to receive was entirely absent. When Jesus's disciples were in need, He was there for them. He gave them food, helped them fish, and He even healed Peter's mother-in-law's fever. They paid Him back by falling asleep at the time of His impending death. Why was God silent in Gethsemane? Why did He allow Jesus to experience abandonment from His friends and those He had helped? Why is God silent when we cry out to Him to save our loved ones? Why is He not there to help when it matters most? Why is God so very silent?

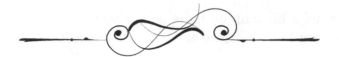

Pierced by God's Silence

As I walk through the hallways of the hospital, everyone sees me as God's representative because of my Dominican habit (the priestly garb). I am often asked, "Please pray for my son or pray for my daughter." Saint Paul says it clearly: "We are therefore Christ's ambassadors, as though God were making his appeal through us" (2 Corinthians 5:20). When I see so many children sick and suffering at the hospital, it makes me cry out to God. I pray for God to show His mercy and love by healing the sick. There are so many patients hooked to huge machines, ECMO, dialysis, feeding tubes, and different monitors. So many IVs are performing one function or another, generating chemical reactions that the body could no longer do on its own. It is a frightening sight to behold. Family members stand in shock when they see their loved ones in that state.

As I walk in and meet the families to pray for patients, I desperately pray for miracles for patients as it is painful to accept that sometimes I also feel God is silent. How can I be a happy ambassador for God when His silence is all we get? It is easy to offer intellectual arguments that God is never silent. "We have to be patient to discern His will in the face of suffering." How can we feel His presence when He is silent in the dark? How can a miracle-working God be silent? That "silence" in our time of need does not imply that God does not care.

Toward the end of the winter season in 2018, I had an incredible experience with a medical doctor. He was a patient going through chemotherapy at the hospital, and he asked me a question that pierced my heart. Why does God choose to be silent when we suffer? Does He not see our tears? This medical doctor had been struggling with a terminal illness. He recounted the sacrifices he had made to become a doctor and achieve his dream of being able to heal others. He was now a patient himself, facing his own fears for the future.

> I grew up in a Christian family and have believed in God all my life. I was taught to have faith in God's goodness and always do things right for the sake of others. When I was diagnosed with pancreatic cancer, I was in shock. I could not understand where that was coming from. I was very angry with myself [and thought] that I must have done something wrong for this to happen. I went to medical school, studied medicine, and later specialized in orthopedics. As I lie down in this hospital bed, I keep asking, God, why are You doing this? I knew I was not supposed to feel that way or question Him, but I could not help it. I was so hopeful that through the prayers offered by my family and faith community, I would heal, but I relapsed. I was angry with God for raising my hopes and abandoning me. I started wondering why He was paying me back with this. I knew I had relapsed in my faith. It was not that I did not believe in God. I never doubted His existence, but for some years, God had not been part of my life. I went to church only when I visited my parents. There was no way I was going to be questioned whether I went to church or not on campus as I always went with them when I came home. On campus, I didn't go because it was not cool. After my wedding, my wife insisted we went to church. I am very happy that I did, and I found God. Now, God and my family are my greatest gifts in life, and I am blessed with three daughters. I somehow saw that God was paying me back with this cancer for those years I had not gone to church or prayed.

I became sick, and sickness taught me more about life than all the textbooks I had read in med school. Yet being in this hospital made me ask questions: Were the years spent studying to be a doctor worth it? All the years of sleeplessness, of doing sixteen-hour shifts at the hospital, of moving from one surgery to another—was all that in vain? What was the value in that? For years, I had stood in the trauma unit tired and burnt out, tending to patients desperate to survive after being involved in automobile accidents. What use were my certificates and years of labor as I am now on this bed with all these needles plunged into me? What opportunities for making memories with my family did I miss? How many holidays did I give up to be at the hospital instead of being on vacation with the family that I love dearly? Was that "chasing after the wind," as Ecclesiastes calls it (Ecclesiastes 1:14)?

Here I am, lying down on my sick bed dying. I ask God, Where are You now? Are You here in the midst of the unimaginable suffering and pain I am enduring? I know You are good, but are You incapable or unwilling to help me? Where is Your love now that it matters most to me? Why do You choose to be silent? Why call upon You if You are not listening? How many other patients have been on this same bed filled with hope, expectations, and the dream of being healed, yet died? Did You hear them as they prayed to You for healing? How many tears, how much anguish and sorrow have these walls, this paint, this ceiling, these lights, and desks heard or seen as they stood as inert witnesses to their suffering?

God, Your silence is what is most infuriating to me. Say something! Show me something! Let me know You are there! Why the silence! That is not fair! Silence, you aggravate the weight of my suffering. Silence, you make the feeling of abandonment even more cruel. You make my darkness darker. I am clinging to hope in the expectation that one day I may pull through. I believed that the pouring rain, the lightning and thunder of this disease and its treatments, would take a toll on me, but that the sun would shine again. I hoped that your light would dispel this darkness. I prayed that one day, everything would be okay again and that all my pain and suffering would not have been in vain. I have researched, studied, prayed and tried to make sense of all this suffering. You have filled my hope with emptiness. God, all I meet is silence. Silence! Absolute silence! That is terrifying.

Living with uncertainty is traumatic for me. I do not know what lies ahead for me. That is incredibly scary. I am not in charge of what is happening to me. Yet I am no longer afraid of dying. But it is so disconcerting to be here at the hospital and not have answers. I look at my medical results, and I dare hope that they will be okay, but they are not. I want to be here to look after my daughters and be there for my wife, but that does not seem a reality. When people come in to speak to me, I can actually see their accelerated heartbeats through their clothes because they have heard that I am a doctor. They are afraid of not saying or doing the right thing. I tell them, "It's okay. I am not a doctor right now. I am the patient."

That is why sharing this moment with You, Father, has been grace-filled. It has given me a different perspective on beauty. I am no longer the teacher in the classroom—I am being taught by life itself. We are all broken and hurting. I am no longer sitting down in the library reading or with my eyes fixated on the computer screen, looking at particles of electrons. I am reading the faces of living beings. I am hearing the sounds and seeing the colors that surround me in my room. I feel the healing hands laid upon me every day. Beauty and my blessings lie in opening my heart daily to the abundance of grace in God and not in my limitations. I am no longer able to write and do all the things I want. Till my last breath, I will express my gratitude to anyone entering my room by saying, "Thanks for your willingness to do your best by being an angel of healing."

As I listened to the doctor in silence, I felt the reality of the pain and anguish he was carrying in his being. It broke my heart, and I was at a loss for words. How does one find grace in this darkness? All I could think of while listening to this doctor was that deafening silence of God. Why is God silent in our suffering? Is He deliberately quietly watching the sorrow caused by trauma, accidents, terrible diseases, the mortification of barrenness, the pain of loneliness and abandonment, suicides, poverty, and all forms of suffering? Is God blind to these things? We continue to ask, Why does He not do anything to stop all of that? The psalmist articulates this anguish when he says:

I cried out to God for help; I cried out to God to hear me. When I was in distress, I sought the Lord; at night I stretched out untiring hands, and I would not be comforted. I remembered you, God, and I groaned; I meditated, and my spirit grew faint. You kept my eyes from closing; I was too troubled to speak. I thought about the former days, the years of long ago; I remembered my songs in the night. My heart meditated and my spirit asked: "Will the Lord reject forever? Will he never show his favor again? His unfailing love vanished forever? Has his promise failed for all time? Has God forgotten to be merciful? Has he in anger withheld his compassion?" (Psalm 77: 1–9)

So it is difficult to understand the principles we can apply to "defend" God in His business of being silent while we suffer as His children. There are so many people who are going through torment and hours of darkness without any hope in their lives. Millions of people cry out to God for help in their distress and anguish. Unfortunately, all they get is silence. It is frustrating in that moment to be seen as being an ambassador to a silent God who is not ready to help His children. It is difficult to stand by this doctor and listen to him talk about his hopes, prayers offered up by his loved ones, and seeing that hope crushed. As a priest, I still get chills as I think of God's silence when I stand bedside to people who are dying. Am I an ambassador of death leading them to heaven (by performing Last Rites to get them ready for heaven), or am I standing with them to bring life and hope?

It is a horrible experience when we pray for healing, and healing doesn't come. When that happens, we feel abandoned, and our hope in God dwindles. We look at ourselves in the mirror and ask, When will this ever end? Are we going to live life like this forever? When will God's promises be fulfilled? At times, we feel miserable because we should have known more and trusted God more, and we should not have doubted. Only when someone has walked in our shoes that we feel they understand our struggle to keep our faith in God alive.

Our Sacrifices Are Never in Vain

As the doctor questioned how worthwhile those sacrifices had been, both in school and at work, we see that we bear the fruit of grace by serving others. "I have been crucified with Christ. It is no longer I who live, but Christ who lives in me, and the life I now live in the flesh I live by faith in the Son of God, who loved me and gave himself for me" (Galatian 2:20). When we share in Christ's suffering, we allow his grace to pour forth from us onto others. Those we touch daily through the little things we do will be blessed. We share in Christ's suffering by making those sacrifices. We may not always see it, but no matter how little our deeds may appear, we are making a difference in our world. Those deeds are what matter most.

The acts of kindness and the sacrifices made to make a difference in our world cannot be quantified monetarily. Each one of us is a gift to our family and to the world. Much like the physician who had sacrificed time and resources to be able to heal others and had now been stricken by disease, we have a purpose. We truly do not have a detailed account of the sacrifices needed to fulfill that purpose. Jesus says, "Enter by the narrow gates."

The value of the treasure we have received is unquantifiable. The number of years that the physician had dedicated to his schooling does not really matter because ignorance is more expensive than knowledge. We miss the point if we focus on the output before we make the sacrifice. No one knows what awaits us tomorrow. What is important is that we are an agent of grace for one another. It is for us to open our eyes and use God's graces to become who we are called to be. So every second spent perfecting God's given gifts to build our community matters. The sacrifices made each and every day in our respective fields matter because of the way they affect our world. Life is not only about us and our personal gain, for we will come and go. The sacrifices we make to help others find meaning in their lives is more precious than money. That is the treasure that endures. "But godliness with contentment is great gain, for we brought nothing into the world, and we cannot take anything out of the world" (1 Timothy 6:6–7).

I reminded the doctor that those years of sacrifice are indeed of tremendous value. Honestly, so much suffering could obscure this value. We are an unquantifiable gift to one another in so many ways that we may not see or notice. So many children would have been left orphaned had he not assisted a mother or father who was involved in a serious accident. Many children would have had serious issues had he not been there to repair their bones. He was their angel of healing and shared the graces he had received. "Blessed is the man who remains steadfast under trial, for when he has stood the test, he will receive the crown of life, which God has promised to those who love him" (James 1:12).

Beneath the surface is the depth of grace present in darkness. God is the only one that can invite himself to partake in the abundance of grace dwelling in the darkness of his reality. That space is sacred and messy, but grace adds fragrance to the messy space so that we encounter beauty in the sacred mess. It is only through the lens of grace that fear is conquered and we experience beauty and peace. This doctor, who was now a patient, had to give himself permission to open his heart to grace. We were taught that it is not right to be angry with God, but what *is* right about being stricken with cancer? Jesus lamented at the cross and cried out to God, "My God, My God, why have You abandoned me?" (Matthew 27:46). If Jesus could say that, why is it that when we anguish, we feel it is not our right to say the same?

Silence as a Springboard to Explore Suffering

In 2017, I read Shusaku Endo's book entitled *Silence* and watched the movie directed by Martin Scorsese. I wish to use it as springboard to explore God's silence in suffering. In this historical fiction, Endo described the life of three Jesuit priests and the sacrifices they made while evangelizing in Japan during the seventeenth century. Like many others who had sacrificed their lives for their faith, they endured persecution at its worst and felt the pain of God's silence.

These missionary priests were forced to watch the members of their flock being tortured and murdered and had to wrestle with the decision to denounce God to save them or remain faithful to God. They were, by all accounts, heroic in their faith, evangelization, and actions, but the trauma of watching the suffering of those with whom they had come to share their faith broke them. Should they have stood watching those who lovingly called them *padre* be slaughtered solely to prove the strength of their faith? Were they overwhelmed by compassion, mercy, and love?

Sebastian Rodrigues showed his devotion to his faith by making the sign of the cross upon his death, which speaks to the fact that the authorities could destroy his body, but they could not destroy his faith in Jesus Christ. The symbolism of holding the cross while dying represents to me the indomitable power of his faith. They crushed his psyche and his body, but his heart remained in Christ. William Wallace, Mel Gibson's character in *Braveheart*, said, "They may take our lives, but they'll never take our freedom." As "padres" to these peasants, how many fathers would not have done whatever it took to save the lives of their children? How many parents would be comfortable watching their children being slaughtered in their presence because they wanted to be heroes? It is true, they will all go to heaven, but it takes extra grace to watch such horror happen to those we love. The challenge presented in *Silence* made me see a higher glory in suffering. Accepting silence and compassion may be more valuable than repeating what we have been taught to say. In theory, words can sound appropriate and wonderful; but when it comes to real situations, they may not necessarily be what is needed.

The Incongruity of Silence

Silence can be unnerving. Silence makes people uncomfortable. How many times have we felt compelled to "fill the void" when someone does not engage in conversation? When we suffer loneliness and abandonment, we long to hear someone's voice. It is devastating to experience God's silence. When a patient is at the hospital, loneliness can create room for a sense of rejection and worthlessness. After visiting hours are over, many patients have nothing but time to feel God's silence and the silence of friends and family members who failed to visit.

> My tears have become my bread, by night, by day, as I hear it said all the day long: "Where is your God?" (Psalm 42:3)

When a loving God who is all powerful does not help us when we need Him most, it is hard to feel His presence. Every unanswered prayer leads us to rely on things of this world. That is why we tend to trust the doctors and medicine instead of depending on a God who seems silent in our darkest hours. We find ourselves asking the same question Jesus's disciples asked when their boat was sinking and Jesus remained asleep. "Teacher, don't you care if we drown?" (Luke 8:22). Is Jesus really sleeping as His children succumb to the storms of life? Jeremiah's lamentation illustrates it best:

> I am the man who has seen affliction by the rod of the Lord's wrath. He has driven me away and made me walk in darkness rather than light; indeed, he has turned his hand against me again and again, all day long. He has made my skin and my flesh grow old and has broken my bones. He has besieged me and surrounded me with bitterness and hardship. He has made me dwell in darkness like those long dead.
>
> He has walled me in so I cannot escape; he has weighed me down with chains. Even when I call out or cry for help, he shuts out my prayer. He has barred my way with blocks of stone; he has made my paths crooked. Like a bear lying in wait, like a lion in hiding, he dragged me from the path and mangled me and left me without help. He drew his bow and made me the target for his arrows.

He pierced my heart with arrows from his quiver. I became the laughingstock of all my people; they mock me in song all day long. He has filled me with bitter herbs and given me gall to drink. He has broken my teeth with gravel; he has trampled me in the dust. I have been deprived of peace; I have forgotten what prosperity is. So, I say, "My splendor is gone and all that I had hoped from the Lord." I remember my affliction and my wandering, the bitterness and the gall. I well remember them, and my soul is downcast within me. (Lamentations 3:1–20)

I reflect on the meaning of suffering by raising those fundamental questions. My eyes were filled with tears as I opened the scriptures. From the words of Prophet Jeremiah, I glean a new dynamic to my frustration and misery when facing unanswered prayers and God's silence. The passage opened the door to finding grace in horrific suffering. God is saying we must wait. All He wants us to do is listen to Him as He speaks to us even in times of darkness and brokenness. He wants us to know that, for generations, others had experienced that same darkness and that He will rescue us just as He saved them.

It is within the context of Prophet Jeremiah's lamentation that the Lord's promises became clearer to me. He was not promising an easy, safe, clear, and straight path. What He was assuring us was safe landing, not that the path would be smooth. He promised that he would walk with us on the journey. With His presence, a difficult journey would be easier. He said to His children the Israelites, "So do not fear, for I am with you; do not be dismayed, for I am your God. I will strengthen you and help you; I will uphold you with my righteous right hand" (Isaiah 41:10).

We often do not take into consideration that no two individuals are the same. My experience with God and the way another person experiences Him are different. God stays with me in my silence. He does not speak human language. He communicates with me in our very own language. It is only through a personal experience with

God that my voice is heard by Him. The way God tends to my needs is not the same way He tends to others'. The way He answers one person's prayers and shows Himself to them is unique and incomparable. That is the fullness of grace.

The Complexity of God's Silence

God's silence in suffering can be terrifying. Many accounts describe Jesus being intentionally silent in the face of suffering before performing miracles. Why did He do that? Why the silence from the Son of God when He could have prevented or healed those who were suffering? Why did Jesus deliberately ignore the Canaanite woman who cried out to him, "Lord, Son of David, have mercy on me! My daughter is demon-possessed and has suffered terribly." Jesus did not say a word. So His disciples came to Him and urged Him, "Send her away, for she keeps crying out after us" (Matthew 15:21–28). Why did Jesus wait three days before going to Bethany to raise Lazarus from the dead when He could have prevented death altogether?

Expressing our fears, brokenness, and pleading with God are all part of the healing journey we need to embark on without fear of judgment. Sometimes all we need to do is pray. We can tell Jesus about the different situations that are troubling our hearts. Those moments are sacred times of grace—times when we have an intimate encounter with God. It is not uncommon for me to get back from the hospital and go directly to the chapel to cry my heart out in front of God. I have screamed, "Why are You silent while this child who is only five months old is dying? Do You not see his mother's broken heart?" In those sacred moments, I have felt God's grace and peace. He is the one that comforts me. I have felt He was letting me know that He had seen the tears of those families I had prayed for and that He was with them. I know that my prayers are not answered exactly as I want, but I have felt peace knowing that He was there carrying us in the palm of His hand. "See, I have engraved you on the palms of my hands" (Isaiah 49:16).

I still feel that God should see the impact of his silence from our perspective. This silence serves as ammunition for atheists and agnostics to mock our faith. They often ask, If there is an all-powerful and all-knowing God, why doesn't He help children suffering and dying of cancer? Where is His love if He can prevent diseases, disasters, and evils in the world but doesn't? Where is God while humans commit atrocities against one another? Why worship Him instead of taking matters into our own hands?

Experiencing the Magnificence of Silence

Silence creates the space where grace and beauty meet to give birth to love. Silence, grace, pain, and beauty are bound together and are inseparable. The whole encounter with suffering becomes the fullness of grace in beauty. We are able to find the indwelling of beauty even in that silence because it is sacred, and God dwells in that sacred space. It is in the light of grace that the love of God is revealed in silence. Darkness ceases to be the home of pain, but it becomes the home of grace to behold the presence of God. That is the revelation of grace that is only possible through God as a gift that opens our eyes so we can see His ever-so-compassionate presence in times of suffering as he suffers with us. In silence, we experience the magnificent presence of God.

When we are at the hospital, God's grace is already there with us even before we set foot into the room, put on the gown, or lie on the bed. That healing grace is already at work through the cleaners, nurses, and all those who work toward securing our physical healing. That is the blessing and the gift of grace that is already given. When we observe this grace, we realize that God is ever present while we wait for answers in our time of uncertainty and fear. We may not get the exact answers we want, but we feel His presence, which gives us comfort and serenity. God promises that He will protect those who place their trust in Him. He will heal, protect, and provide for His children.

> Because he holds fast to me in love, I will deliver him; I will protect him, because he knows my name. When he calls to me, I will answer him; I

will be with him in trouble; I will rescue him and
honor him. With long life I will satisfy him and
show him my salvation. (Psalm 91:14–16)

Every created thing found in nature interacts with one another.
These interactions create tension, fear, and pain but are also interspersed with joy and happiness. As human beings, we are not protected or insulated from crisis. "For the creation waits in eager expectation for the children of God to be revealed" (Romans 8:19). We
find meaning and peace in times of suffering when we look at things
through the lens of grace. It does not remove the reality of the pain
found in crisis. It simply changes our perspective on the anxiety and
stress we feel. It gives us encouragement and the sense that whatever
we are going through is not in vain. There is magnificent glory hidden and being revealed in suffering.

As Sebastian Rodrigues said in *Silence*, "I do not believe that
God has given us this trial for no purpose. I know that the day will
come when we will clearly understand why this persecution with all
its suffering has been bestowed upon us—for everything that Our
Lord does is for our good." We may never figure out the purpose but
remain hopeful. Saint Peter says, "Beloved, do not be surprised at
the fiery trials when it comes upon you to test you, as though something strange were happening to you. But rejoice insofar as you share
Christ's sufferings, that you may also rejoice and be glad when his
glory is revealed" (1 Peter 4:12–13).

Yet how do we find grace in suffering if we can't hear God?
I believe God's silence is an invitation to encounter Him. I see an
interconnection between God's silence, grace, beauty, pain, suffering, darkness, peace, and serenity in that sacred space of emptiness.
Instead of equating God's silence with neglect and abandonment, I
hear God's voice saying, "You are not alone." I see the suffering of
patients drawing them to an intimate relationship with God.

One of the things we had to learn as children is caution.
Children are free-spirited. They run around without shame, freely
expressing themselves. Grown-ups teach us rules and what is deemed
inappropriate. We comply with rules for fear of repercussion, shame,

or humiliation. We are careful with our words and actions to avoid punishment. Invariably, our spirited voices become silenced. Not so long ago, males were denied the gift of expressing their sorrow with tears because "boys don't cry." In order to avoid shame, men became mute and voiceless. That behavior was perpetuated for many generations. Unfortunately, some men became addicted to loneliness, and many others lost the compassionate heart of a father. We built a generation of human beings that became indifferent The tide has now shifted, and young people fight for the sanctity of every life and focus on a better future for all.

In order to experience the abundance of God's grace found in suffering, we have to embark on a quest to know and understand the source of our suffering. Every generation has searched for answers. What have we been taught about suffering? God has warned us that in our world, we are not immune to suffering. "He causes the sun to rise on the evil and the good, and sends rain on the righteous and the unrighteous" (Matthew 5:45). We are also reminded to "praise God in every situation" (1 Thessalonians 5:18). How does thanking God in the face of unimaginable suffering make sense?

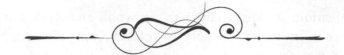

Incomprehensible Euphoria

As a child, growing up in the eastern part of Nigeria, we sang a hymn in the Igbo dialect, *"Chineke di mma."* The meaning of the song is that God the Creator is good. The chorus of the song is simply, *"O di mma,"* which means, "He is good." This song is built on the solid foundation laid by generations of testimony affirming God's goodness. This witness was handed from one generation to another to show that God has been good to us, His children. The gift of life, health, family, friends, shelter, and protection confirm this.

I fear that the stories of disease, violence, war, death, and unimaginable suffering in our world tend to eclipse our appreciation of God's goodness. It is becoming difficult to accept the witness of so many people testifying to these blessings that come from God. When we see so many diseases, sicknesses, and suffering, it hurts. It hurts far more when we, our family members, or our friends are affected. We look up to heaven and ask, "God, are You not here? Are You tired of Your children? Are You no longer interested in reaching out to help those in need?" God may appear distant from our world and from us when we cannot feel His helping hand. However, it is us who keep distancing ourselves from Him. Whereas we lament that electronics have replaced personal interactions, we cannot relinquish our devices. We have become enamored with features that allow us quick access to information but neglected to notice the risk of becoming dependent on it. Simple things that we would have once memorized are abdicated to the phone.

We cannot imagine being without our devices, but we don't seem to mind not having a relationship with God. We tend to forget to give thanks to God for His goodness even though the Bible reminds us, "In everything give thanks: for this is the will of God in

Christ… I will bless the Lord at all times; His praise will always be on my lips" (1 Thessalonians 5:18). "I will bless the Lord at all times, His praise shall continually be in my mouth" (Psalm 34:1).

In the summer of 2017, I had just finished my eight-hour shift at the hospital and was feeling particularly drained. I joined other priests for our evening prayers. The psalm we read that day said, "Give thanks to the Lord for he is good, his love endures forever" (Psalm 107:1). I was awestruck. I had come back with a heavy heart after visiting a patient the same age as me who had been told that her cancer was spreading aggressively. The doctors told her that they were running out of treatment options for her. Even after chemotherapy, radiation, and surgeries, her recent test results showed that her cancer was spreading again. In no uncertain terms, she was told that she would be dying soon. She was basically handed a death sentence.

I watched her tears pouring down like raindrops. I saw the anguish of her family, and my heart wept with theirs. She had hoped she would pull through and had fought so hard with a good resilient spirit. She was willing to risk any new treatment or research trial drugs available. She endured the side effects of every treatment without complaining. She was very positive and believed that God would see her through while she bore her pain. She had now been officially told that her time was short. I was truly heartbroken as I went in for prayers, and the psalm read, "Give thanks to the Lord for He is good."

Listening to this patient telling her story resurrected the fear of not finding God in our darkest moment. Her sister sat at her bedside, trying to act stoic. However, her entire demeanor screamed disappointment and anger with God. The hope that had motivated them to carry on fighting using every treatment option imaginable had not restored her back to health. Like most of us, she had been told we are not supposed to be angry or disappointed with God, let alone show it. However, I saw in the patient's sister quiet sorrow and anguish. She was stunned by the information. I could almost hear her scream in silence, "I am angry even though I know I am not supposed to be. I want to yell, 'God, why are you doing this?' I want to cry, but I don't want to appear weak. I have to be strong for my sister. I want to scream at the top of my lungs, but I am supposed to trust God. I expected a miracle for her."

Although I had prayed this particular psalm more times than I can count over the years, it struck a different chord that evening. After prayers, I went back to my room, and my mind could not stop trying to come up with ways to find God's goodness in suffering. Why on earth, out of every passage in the Scriptures, that was the very one we had right after my experience? I looked up and asked God, "Is this a trick? Why couldn't I find Your love that endures forever while watching her in pain, physically and spiritually broken? Where are You now?"

I was taught not to question God. I was not supposed to feel the way I was feeling that day because we should always place our hope in Him in every circumstance. I could not bear the pain I felt stepping into that space and imagining that I was the one on that bed. I was the one hearing such news. I am not exempt from that. It was scary. In times of suffering, we are always reminded of the story of Job and the need to accept everything as the will of God. We have heard this millions of times when it comes to explaining suffering. Looking at someone my age on the hospital bed dying made it real for me. It could be me any day and anytime. That propelled me to look for answers for her and for myself.

While in the room with the patient and her sister, my heart ached. At that moment, I was overwhelmed by the absurdity of the mystery of suffering. I was heartbroken. None of the theological answers I used to offer in times of suffering seemed sufficient to provide comfort. Once at home, I sat in my room, and my eyes welled up. My entire being was searching for answers, Is God's love eternal? Does God really care for our well-being? Is He in the dark with us? How do we give thanks to the Lord in the midst of such grief? I believe these crosses are not from God, but how do we make sense of His goodness and love in times like these?

There I was, sitting, wrestling with everything I had been taught, and trying to make sense of things as I faced the reality of life. I knew I was supposed to see everything that happens as the will of God. I believe and always knew that nothing happens without God's knowledge. Things happen for a reason as we know, but does God will these things? Yes, I knew there has to be a reason even if we can't comprehend it. But how do I tell that to someone whose only son or daughter is dying at the hospital? It is easy when we preach it, but when that suffering is up close and personal, not so much. I thought to myself, God must have His reasons to allow a little five-year-old child to die of leukemia. I entertained that thought for a few seconds and promptly shouted, "Give me a break! What reason could there be?" No response makes suffering any more bearable. It may help manage the hurt, but the pain in our hearts remains. There has to be something else in suffering that can bring us to grace.

Going back to the young woman whose story I shared, she felt broken after she was told there was nothing else to be done. She was a devout Christian. She tried to do what was right and lived her whole life being faithful to God. She devoted her life to serving God through her church and community. She was a kindergarten teacher, and to her, her students were her children. She was like a mom to each and every one of them. Everyone was a member of her family. She never had children of her own. When it came to children, as a teacher, there was never birth control. Every child was important to her, and they were all treated with dignity and respect. She believed that if given the opportunity to thrive, they would be better children, especially as part of her family. The challenge then was to comprehend why after such dedication and sacrifice, the payback she received was dying in a hospital bed. The doctors put it nicely by saying, "We are running short on treatment options."

The Absurdity of Our Expectations

I have been expected to say, "Thanks be to God," in every situation. This is what we were told and learned over the years. Everyone quotes Saint Paul: "In all things give thanks, for this is God's will" (1 Thessalonians 5:18). This does not work at the hospital when we receive a bad diagnosis. It is, however, possible, after a while, for people to learn from their suffering, transform their pain, and grow. It is disingenuous to expect the initial reaction to being hospitalized to be, "Thanks be to God. I am loving this."

Truth be told, I found it very difficult and uncomfortable to say, "Thank You, God, my friend has cancer." Should I also go to God in prayer after my visit with this patient and say, "Thank You, God, your 19-year-old daughter's cancer is spreading, and there is nothing the doctors can do to help her. She will soon be coming back to You." That is very hard. How do we say, "Thank You, God," for the bad things that God has allowed to come our way? How could we thank God for loneliness, mental illness, and depression? How do we say "thanks be to God" when we are put down and repressed by others? How on earth can we thank God when someone has looked down on us and treated us as if we were not good enough? Is it possible to say "thanks be to God" when our sacrifices and efforts are never appreciated by colleagues, in church, and even by our families? How does one say "thanks be to God" when we fail to find any answers to our prayers? How do we thank God when bad things come our way? Should somebody thank God when they are given the news that they have a chronic and incurable disease? Should people say, "Thank God, I am happy that I am sick and sickness rocks"? That would be glorifying sickness. How do we accept suffering, cope with it, and carry it daily as a cross? It is very hard.

I was walking along the hallway during my first week at the hospital, and when I was about to enter a room, a nurse approached me and said, "Father, thank God you are here. The patient you are coming to see just received the worst news of her life. She has a bad liver, and she was told she has a few days to live. Another doctor will be coming in to speak with her soon." I was in shock because of the directness of the message. I walked in and greeted the woman. A doctor walked in and explained her medical condition to her. In summary, he told her, "Due to the nature of your condition, you only have thirty-two hours to live. Is there anything else I can help you with?" Seriously? "No! Thanks."

I stood there as the doctor left agitated and visibly upset. My head was spinning. I wanted to run out of the room, down the stairs, and straight home. I could not imagine being told, "You have thirty-two hours to live." That only happens in movies, not in real life. What could I do in this situation? I was right there when she received such a devastating prognosis. The woman cried, and I was with her partaking in that pain. I opened my mouth to speak, but nothing came out. There was nothing I could say that would make sense. Tears flowed from my eyes. I pulled a chair closer, sat, and just cried with her. After a long time, I asked her if her family was aware of her condition. She said they didn't know and that everything had been very sudden as she came for a checkup and was sent to do more tests. I just sat with her in shock.

Later, I told her, "If what the doctor said is true, maybe you should prepare yourself. Invite your family and give them your blessing. I know you talked about your granddaughter. Maybe it would bring healing to her to receive blessings from you as they also bless you. This is devastating news, and time is not on your side." It was painful but beautiful to see the family gathered around her the next day. She told them, "Thank God the priest was here when I got the news. There was no way I could have processed this on my own. He was God sent. I can now say that I am ready no matter what happens." She was able to bless her granddaughter and family. She thanked me profusely. We prayed with her, and I did the Last Rites with her entire family present. She died within the time she had been told she had left. In this situation, my presence as a priest was comforting. No medical explanation could have helped her to make sense of her circumstance. Yet I was broken inside because how does one remain positive and thankful to God under these conditions?

In this instance, when do I start to say, "Thank You, God"? The fact is that we do not jump to say thank-you for "gifts" we do not appreciate. If we ever do, it is to avoid offending the giver's sensibilities. When it comes to something we vehemently dislike or would cause us harm, we flat-out reject it. We would never deliberately accept a snake that we knew would kill us. Therefore, it is difficult to thank God for things we dread and hate, like being sick. Any human being could become sick on any given day, and no insurance could protect anyone from that. That does not mean that people should wish the worst to happen to them. When adverse things happen, we lose all control. The only comfort we may find is the realization that certain things are beyond our human comprehension. We do whatever we can and trust God with the rest.

Looking around at our world, how do we make sense of the belief that the love of God endures forever? We live in a world filled with crippling poverty and unspeakable suffering. Each one of us, in one way or another, witnesses the cruelty and criminality prevalent in our world. We have directly or indirectly witnessed the human capacity to inflict pain on those who are vulnerable. How do we find God's goodness even as the power of evil in our world has tripled? How do we explain the horrifying atrocities that man commits against one another? These hardships and painful reality becloud God's goodness.

I remember the story of Saint Theresa of Avila, a Carmelite nun in sixteenth-century Spain. She is one of the great saints because of her commitment and devotion to God in prayer and a life of poverty. One of the stories told of her was that she was traveling through rugged roads. Her saddle slipped, and she found herself under the belly of the donkey as they were passing a stream. She complained to the Lord, and she heard the reply: "Theresa, whom the Lord loves, He chastises. This is how I treat all my friends." She replied, "No wonder You have so few."

The drive to find comfort in times of suffering is the gift of grace.

Part II

THE MYSTERY

As you do not know the path of the wind, or how the body is formed in a mother's womb, so you cannot understand the work of God, the Maker of all things (Ecclesiastes 11:5).

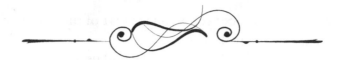

The Dazzling Mystery of Grace

Mysterium tremendum et fascinans (mystery that is fascinating yet terrifying).

When we are hospitalized, it is not only stressful but exhausting. The pain, the sleepless nights, the talking, and annoying voices in the hallways could be irritating. The crown jewel of this experience is the uncertainty prior to receiving test results. Those reports from the doctors are unpredictable and could be scary. When I speak to patients at the hospital, I encourage them to hope for the best and trust their doctors. In reality, it is easier said than done. The hospital is an intimidating place for virtually every patient and family member. The reality is that no patient goes to the hospital because they want to. It is not a Holiday Inn. They are there because they have to be, and that is why it is frightful.

How do we then get to the level of grace that allows us to see everything in our lives as a grace? It is possible when we put all our trust in God by accepting our human nature, and we open ourselves up to becoming better? Acknowledging the presence of grace at all times would mean that we understand that in every situation, God is with us. God does not tell us His plans in advance; He reveals them gradually. I recently saw a quote in Pinterest, "If God showed you all He has planned for you, it would boggle your mind. If you could see the doors He is going to open, the opportunities that will cross your path, and the people who will show up, you would be so amazed, excited, and passionate that it would be very easy to set your mind for victory. This is what faith is all about. You have to believe it before you see it. God's favor is surrounding you like a shield. Every setback is a setup for a comeback. Every bad break, every disappointment, and every person who does you wrong is part of the plan to get you to where you are supposed to be."

God does not tell us His plans. If he told us everything that will happen in our lives from beginning to end, we would not have free will. We would be like robots programmed to do what we were made to do. If that were the case, we wouldn't love someone because we felt it; we would do it because we were conditioned to do it. That is not what God wants from us. God is journeying with us, and that is the grace that sustains us in the most terrible and difficult experiences. That is what makes the difference in our lives and it means that grace is mysterious.

The Sophistication of Grace

I recall first hearing about grace in church. When I was learning the catechism of the Catholic church in the Igbo language (Igbo is the language spoken in the eastern part of Nigeria where I was born and grew up), *grace* was translated as "grasia." In my first interview to enter the seminary, I was asked to explain the meaning of *grace*. I told the interview board that "grace is the supernatural gift that God gives us as a favor, the revealing light of a deep *grasia* [I used the Igbo word] that helps us to have strong faith without placing our thoughts on whatever God is revealing." When I finished giving this answer, the vocation director asked me, "Were you translating from Igbo?" *Yes!* That was what I knew. I knew I had messed up because they were all laughing. I had a good laugh at myself too.

Grace is a familiar word that each of us has probably heard over a million times. People answer to the name *Grace*. It is in our everyday vocabulary and conversations. It is not only my dialect that struggles with finding words that could explain the meaning of the word *grace*. When I talk about grace here, what do I mean? Most of us grew up learning that grace is a favor, that it is an unmerited, undeserved, and unearned gift from God. In the book of Luke, Mary was approached by the angel Gabriel, who said, "Hail Mary, full of grace," and some translations have it as "highly favored." There have been so many theological discussions and books written to explore the intricacies of grace. The essence of grace lies in its inherent mystery. No human language can fully express its rich meaning. While experiencing grace for ourselves, grace becomes the teacher of what *grace* means. That takes the conversation to, how do we experience grace for ourselves?

Mary, the mother of Jesus, was full of grace. If we translate *grace* as "highly favored," where do we find God's favor as she ran to Egypt for safety after the birth of her son? Where was the favor as for three days she anxiously and tearfully searched for her son? How was she highly favored when she had to see her son being persecuted by the Pharisees? Was she highly favored while watching the body of her son at the foot of the cross? What if there were more to grace than favor? What if this unmerited gift could sometimes be a favor and others like a rose full of thorns? Let's suppose that grace is a gift given to everyone that may or may not be deserved. Could this be an undeserved gift given to us by God to become better children of God?

To understand the meaning of *grace*, I feel there are many layers, ambiguities, and a lack of clarity that need to be addressed as we try to determine what grace is. Grace can only be experienced to be understood. My experiences with grace have taught me that grace is part of the human fiber. I still lament that my Catholic childhood did not help me understand grace because it was always in competition with sin. We had to go to confession to be "in a state of grace." This model allows for the thought that there are times when God's grace leaves us because of sin. When we commit a mortal sin, grace leaves, and we are without grace. If we commit a venial sin, we still have some grace, but sin is fighting to separate us from God. This idea would imply that grace is something we merit because we have to be holy to keep it.

Grace is therefore more than what we thought. It has multiple layers that are quite hard to fully comprehend. There are many people who may feel they already understand it. Grace is forever unfolding. The concept of it being an unmerited and undeserved favor is true. However, it is not the whole story because grace is still embedded in whatever God is revealing. Waiting for what God is trying to reveal is unsettling. The gift is dependent on the giver, and God is the giver. Whatever He gives us, even when we do not understand or want it, is enveloped by grace. It is very hard to call suffering a favor from God. We must remain steadfast no matter what God reveals through the graces He pours onto us through suffering. We tend to forget about the unpredictability of grace. We think of grace as those moments when we are not stressed by problems, worries, and everything is seemingly going as planned.

To define *grace* just as a favor limits the definition of *grace*. Each one of us experiences grace even when we are not aware of it. Grace dwells in unfamiliar places. If only we were able to see that beyond the stars lies the darkness of the night. Without darkness, the stars would be undistinguishable. To see those stars in the dark without a sense of guilt or shame is my definition of grace. Grace is therefore that exploration, the search and discovery of the abundance of grace in the darkest moments of our lives. It is the unending hunger and search to find meaning and authenticity in the midst of suffering. It is that passion to wait and listen in silence to see the beauty of the gifts God has bestowed upon us in abundance. The gift of humanness as we await salvation. All these little stars represent God's graces sparkling in our lives beyond the darkness of suffering.

Grace is not a story with a happy ending. The end and the beginning are not clearly discernible; neither are they distinguishable. While at the hospital, I feel that God changes the goalpost whenever I feel I am ahead. Just as I was starting to feel that I understood God, grace, and how to be a good child of God, the post shifts. Grace is the gift that allows us to embrace our dependence on God. It is to purposefully place our trust in him instead of on ourselves. Grace is to understand that we don't have all the answers and to be okay with it. It is the ability to see grace as we start again. Grace is being plagued by suspense, unpredictability, uncertainty, and yet embracing the experience. Grace dwells in the secret beauty being revealed. It is terrifying to be in that dark without realizing that God's grace dwells there.

Jesus is the example of the fullness of grace. From the moment of his birth, Jesus went about sharing the grace of God with those in need of that grace. At birth, He chose to be born among sheep and other animals. Quite often, the beauty of the Christmas manger fails to depict the hardship in Jesus's birth. We see the beautiful decorations and lights shining on the crib, and we forget the smell of manure and the harshness of the conditions. Jesus still allowed Himself to start His life in this humble setting and lived his life in that spirit until the end. For this reason, he became a refugee in Egypt until Herod, who tried to kill him, was dead. So He knew the struggles, the fears, and the pain of being a foreigner in another country. He suffered the uncertainty of the future with them. Instead of remaining with the learned and the teachers of the law, He left them to be with fishermen. He chose to be with fraudsters like Zacchaeus and went to their homes to feast with them. Everyone in the community knew Zacchaeus was a sinner, and Jesus still chose to be with him. Did Jesus know Judas Iscariot as well? Why did Jesus include him as one of his disciples? He was a thief and had stolen from the treasury. Although Jesus was aware of the secret activities of Judas Iscariot, he never set a trap to catch him, never accused him, or shamed him. He knew he was a cheat and weak but still chose him to be one of His disciples.

Jesus's grace was evident when He chose to be with those who were struggling with their imperfections. He did not cast them away. He accepted Matthew just as he was, a tax collector. He did not force him to change before He received him as His disciple. He chose to stay with the woman at the well and spent His whole day talking to her. Apparently, He followed her to the village to preach to others. This was considered taboo in Israel at the time. That a young Jewish man would be seen with a woman, who had had five husbands and the one she was living with was not even her husband, and a Samaritan no less, was unconscionable. He was, however, not afraid of giving Himself grace to be with her despite being mocked. Jesus was a friend to Mary Magdalene. He did not hide His appreciation for her and deemed her a blessing. He accepted her gift of a special expensive ointment for His burial. Jesus is therefore our model for what grace is, as manifested by His association with widows, the demonized, the rejected, alcoholics, criminals, and all those who were sick and suffering. Jesus never forced the Pharisees, who believed themselves to be grace-filled, to accept Him. He gave them the opportunity to share in this grace, although they closed their hearts to it.

Grace Unfolds

Grace is found when the unexpected happens. It is allowing ourselves to accept that predictability is a myth. There are times when we understand things, but sometimes nothing makes sense. There may be moments during our search for meaning when we find our answers and exclaim, "Wow!" At that very moment, we see grace in its plenitude and in abundance. There may be times when the meaning simply eludes us. We still see those moments as grace. Life does not just happen when we have the perfect gift of grace, when everything is moving forward as we envisioned. Grace can be found when we are open to living with uncertainty and with the reality that things can change at any given moment. The abundance of grace is manifested when we find ourselves at peace, doing our best no matter what is going on at the time and regardless of how scary it may be. That is the gift Jesus brings to the table. He wants us to realize that in those times of fear, there is grace. He would not abandon us because He is the God of compassion who suffers with us. Being open to that reality is the gift of grace. This is an uncommon gift.

Why didn't God shield Jesus from suffering? Why didn't He protect Jesus from the hands of the Pharisees and Sadducees, and from Pilate and all the injustices He had to endure? Why did God allow His Son to be a symbol of injustice instead of protecting Him? Why should God allow Herod to butcher innocent children to protect His own child while so many women had to live the rest of their lives in anguish without their sons? Why did God allow His Son to carry the cross and endure suffering throughout His life? Grace, therefore, is not as simple as we assume it to be. There are so many aspects to it that it is only by grace that we do see grace.

The Unpredictability of Grace

One Sunday after Mass, I went to the hospital for my visitation. I met a patient who was undergoing dialysis at the hospital. He was always in good spirits and had a positive energy. That day, he was downcast. He said, "Father, why is God like this? The truth is, I no longer feel His presence in this hospital bed. I have been struggling with my kidneys all these years, and I have learned to deal with it. Last week, I had a test and was told that there may be a tumor in my stomach. When I received this bad news from the doctors, it was difficult for me to see that God was with me in this abyss. This really sucks. I feel deflated and discouraged. I feel frustrated with God right now. Even when I raise my eyes up to Him, I cannot feel His presence."

It is heartbreaking to be in this type of situation. Even with limitations, he had been able to find comfort. He was positive and hopeful, and I was able to see that as grace. What if grace were also present when things turn the way we did not expect? What if we need to start searching for grace even in the darkest times of life? This is the challenge we face when enduring suffering. Prolonged suffering is a challenge and a great source of distress for anyone going through it. There is that hope that lets us carry on. We figure that there has to be a lesson to be learned from our situation. This could be a source of comfort and strength in difficulty. Our hearts are comforted when we think there is a higher purpose to our suffering. It allows us to continue and not give up. We may never know why we suffer as we do, but the sense of a higher purpose helps fan the flames of hope that keep our hearts on fire. A little glimpse of hope helps us bear the cross. It is quite devastating to experience hope only to be faced with yet another setback. This is what leads to despair and hopelessness and resurrects the fundamental question—*why*? We all have our stories and experiences with things that make us scream the question, "God, why?" Whether it affects us directly or not, the reality of pain and sickness stares us right in the face. It is just a reality we cannot escape.

God is always at work and makes His presence be felt when we least expect it. A woman became very distressed when she saw my chaplain badge while at the emergency department waiting room. She started shouting, "What is the chaplain doing here? What are you people not telling me?" I smiled and walked to her. I explained to her that when someone is admitted to the hospital as a trauma patient, the medical team takes care of that person. The chaplain is there to help guide the family by telling them where to wait, what to do next, and by being a source of comfort to them. This saves doctors time and allows them to focus on patients instead of having to deal with family members. When the medical team is ready, the chaplain takes the family around to see the patient. If they ask for prayer, the chaplain prays with them, or he prays silently asking for healing. In a way, the chaplain could be seen as the liaison between the family and the medical team. In times of emergency, there is acute anxiety, and everyone present is plagued by uncertainty. The woman relaxed after my explanation and was at peace. While waiting for the doctors, we started a conversation.

"You are a chaplain?"

"Yes."

"I am angry with God."

"How so?"

"I always believed that God cared. Looking back at everything that my family has gone through in the past few years, it is difficult to think that God cares. I am struggling to go to church these days. Where on earth was God when my grandson was hit by a truck? He was driving home for Thanksgiving, and our entire family was waiting for him to arrive. Next thing we know, we get a call from the state police telling us that we needed to go over to the emergency department at the hospital. My grandson died a few weeks later at the hospital. That call shattered our joy, Thanksgiving celebration, and our world. Nobody touched the turkey that had been roasting in the oven for hours. The potatoes on the stove, fresh fruits, salad, gravy, and desert were all left behind and ended up in the trash. The turkey remained in the freezer for more than two years before it was tossed. I am still hurting and broken by the pain of that loss. I find it hard to believe that God is there when He allowed something like that to happen to us. The chaplain was there that day and helped us. Here I am again, dealing with this, and the chaplain shows up. That is why I was terrified."

Suffering hurts, but giving in to despair is dangerous. We can be tormented by the pain and fear we experience. To carry the cross is never easy. We have to see that God is with us and listen to the story He is telling us during our journey. I don't necessarily understand the mystery of why God does what He does, especially in times of suffering. Before now, I thought I understood suffering. I am sorry to humbly say, "I don't understand."

I went into the trauma bay to see how the patient was doing. I stood in shock when I saw he was dead. I was horrified as I looked at his lifeless body. He was flown in by helicopter when he was found on the road after having jumped from the overpass. He was brought in unresponsive but with the hope that something could be done to help. Everything that could be done was done to save him, but to no avail. How do I go back again to this woman to tell her to see the grace of God in all of this? I couldn't bear to be with the doctors as they gave her the sad news, but I had to be. I seriously wanted to run away and go home. How could this woman find comfort and consolation from God again after this experience? I prayed and wept with her as she stayed at the hospital. The excruciating pain of this news was heartbreaking. It was horrible to be a chaplain that day. I sat with this woman till other family members came, and we prayed.

I was praying to be able to find grace in that dark hour. Where does one find comfort when everything seems lost? "He heals the broken-hearted and binds up their wounds" (Psalm 147:3). What God is offering me daily is to see glimpses of grace in the broken pieces of our daily lives. He invites us to open our eyes and heart to see that he is with us, has always been, and will continue to be with us. He has not given up on us yet. He is sharpening us through those terrifying experiences. We must open our hearts to know what He is trying to say to us. The Lord says His faithfulness never ceases. He uses His own logic and His own language. That is why our understanding is limited as we search to understand God through our limited brain and resources. The grace we seek is to remain steadfast in times of trials and difficulties. We pray for the grace to see that God is there with us even on that rocky road. "The Lord is close to the broken-hearted, and saves those who are crushed in spirit" (Psalm 34:18).

How do we find the grace of abundance to live in the moment and appreciate the gifts of today while investing in the future? How do we build our lives and connect grace between yesterday, today, and tomorrow? How do we remind ourselves that the graces of today are inseparable from the trials endured yesterday and the foundation to learn to avoid pitfalls tomorrow? How to see the dangers of tomorrow and, at the same time, appreciate the gift of hope tomorrow could bring? We live today in a constant vortex of grace, learning, growth, fear, tension, gratitude, desire while placing our hope in tomorrow's bliss.

To find this grace in the darkest hours of our lives, we must learn to open our hearts to God's revelation even in suffering. This learning is invaluable. Without learning, suffering becomes meaningless and will only lead to despair. Learning from suffering is what transforms our brokenness. It is the foundation for a new life and growth. When our suffering is not transformative, we become choked, crushed, and it could lead to despair. For this transformation to happen, we have to unlearn, relearn, and reclaim our lost childlike innocence. It is this relearning that allows us to transform pain into a grace-filled experience.

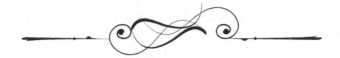

An Allegory

Once upon a time, there was a hunter who became very rich overnight. Nobody in the community knew the source of his unexpected wealth. With his money, he rebuilt his house, bought land and horses. Everyone in his village wanted to know his secret. The community speculated day and night on the source of his sudden riches. "He must have discovered a treasure," they said. "He must have killed an elephant and sold it," retorted others. He heard all their gossip but remained silent. He only told them that his treasures came from a cave. The villagers wanted to know the location of the cave. He was monitored day and night to ensure he would not sneak out at night to go back to the cave.

The hunter was always at home. He refused to go back to hunting. He said it was a journey that he had made once and would rather not repeat. He helped the poor in his village, built houses for widows, and sent food to the sick. These acts of charity were not enough for the villagers as they wanted more from him. They wanted to go to the cave themselves to retrieve their share of the riches and did not hide their contempt for him. One day, while walking along the road back from the market, he was accosted by two women.

"So you refuse to share the source of your wealth with others? You are very selfish, greedy, and covetous. You want to remain the only rich man in the village so every other person continues to serve you."

The second friend continued, "You want us to bow to you for money instead of showing us where to find ours. You are promoting yourself so everyone will respect you. You are not generous at all. You are doing everything for your own glory."

They disparaged him and laughed at him as he silently walked on without raising his head until he got to his house. This experience was constant, and many children mocked and laughed at him when they passed by him. For some weeks, the villagers hoped that the hunter would reveal his secret cave, but after some months, their hope dwindled. As years went by, the hope for a revelation vanished, and everyone was left with only memories of the stories. When the man got old, he decided to share the location of his secret cave.

The men and women in the community gathered and thanked the hunter for deciding to reveal his secret. They pleaded, "Forgive us for our contempt and pride. We were mean to you all these years, and we are sorry for that. We are sorry for the children who mocked you." The old hunter accepted their apology. They held a meeting to choose seven young men to go to this cave. These young men were very proud and happy they had been chosen to retrieve the treasures.

The old hunter warned them, "The journey you want to embark on will be arduous. It will be a seven-day journey. The roads are treacherous and daunting. Night and day, you will traverse many forests and swim across rivers. You have to be aware that you will go through dangerous villages. The rain in the forest will be harsh and destructive, and the thunderstorms will be severe."

He paused and looked at them in the eye. "Expect deadly animals and poisonous snakes to attack you. Some of you may die during the quest. This will be a dangerous adventure because of the risk involved. If you get there, you will find the cave and the treasure inside. If you wish to change your mind, I would not blame you."

With this information, the seven brave men set out with enthusiasm. They were aware of the possibility of danger, but were not deterred by the old hunter's warnings. They said goodbye to their families and friends as they received their blessings. The villagers watched them with excitement as they left with the hunter's map in search for the cave and treasures. They didn't care about the rain, the sun, poisonous snakes, terrifying animals, or any discomfort they could experience. The hope of getting to the cave and coming back with treasures was worth the sacrifice. As they traveled, they discussed their plans for when they got back. One said he was going to build a new house for his mother, and another said he hoped to marry his girlfriend. The third expressed his bitterness because the most beautiful girl in the village had refused him. "Now she will beg me to marry her," he quipped. Another said the first thing he hoped to do was have a banquet and feast with friends and family.

On their third day of this journey through the forest, they suddenly heard a sound. "Silence!" They stood frozen with fear! Scanning the trees, the bushes, the dead branches, and the leaves, they waited silently. The expression on their faces was enough to communicate with one another without any sound, and their eyes displayed the look of terror. They listened in horror and trepidation at the rustling sound of the leaves. They waited to see where the sound had originated. With the leaves rapidly and persistently fluttering, they knew something was terribly wrong. It was quite obvious that they had company in the forest. Like a flash, a leopard jumped on one of them. They fought it vigorously and killed it. Unfortunately, the young man who was attacked by the leopard was bitten on the neck, and he bled to death. They were in shock and cried as they mourned the young man's death. After a while, they garnered courage and continued on their journey. They walked for miles and were tired, but they had been warned of the danger of resting. They continued with increased fear.

While on their journey, they heard another strange noise. This time, it was a hissing sound. Before they could check what was happening, they saw a huge snake. It was a poisonous snake. It launched a vicious and unexpected attack against another young man. The strike delivered a lethal dose of venom. They killed the snake, but unfortunately, the poison had already entered the young man's bloodstream, causing his leg to swell. He was paralyzed, and they laid him down. Suddenly other parts of his body started to swell too. They were horrified as they watched him convulse and die. One of them vomited after having witnessed this. They were terrified and could not continue on the journey. The guy who hoped to have a banquet when he got home insisted, "I must go back. My life is more important than these treasures. I think it is important for us to go back alive."

"You were always a weakling. I always wondered why you were even chosen in the first place. We were chosen because they felt we were man enough. Going back would be the equivalent to failing our families and friends, who placed their trust in us. We have to continue," the young man whom the beautiful girl had refused sternly commanded.

Someone else said, "I think it may even be too late to try to go back from here because we could still face those same dangers on the way back. Maybe we should have returned after the first attack. Now we may have to continue."

They reluctantly continued on their journey. While they walked, there was this luxurious luscious smell. They paused, stopped walking, looking around there before them was the largest unimaginable bunch of fleshly ripe wild blueberries. The blueberries stood there delightfully appealing that they forgot everything going on and enjoyed the delicious juicy taste. After this, they happily went on.

As they kept going, the person walking in front stepped on a trap. He was lifted up to the treetop, and a spear pierced his heart. He died instantly as blood gushed from his body. They trembled at the sight of this and felt dead themselves. This experience killed their hope for survival and their chances of making it back alive. They sat there and sobbed.

"Is this how our lives are to end? Why did the old hunter send us into the forest to be slaughtered like this? We were not the only ones who were mean to him, so why did he do this to us? Why did he send us on this suicide mission? Our blood is more precious than any treasure."

In tears, the young man hoping to marry the beautiful girl lamented, "Maybe it is my fault. We should have started heading back immediately. What is the use if we are not alive to share the treasure? Is this how we will all die?"

Feeling powerless and hopeless, they all sat down. Looking up, the guy accused of being lazy asserted, "Look, there in the front is a striking blueish wild flower blooming in the midst of these dried fallen leaves. Our hope for survival is never to give up. It is late. We have no option now but to move on. Let's go because if we stay, we are already dead. At least we should put up a fight before we die."

While these young men were experiencing these traumatic events, the villagers started quarrelling with one another.

"When the treasure arrives, we should have a party and celebrate for a week. We should tell everyone to start practicing for the dance." "We should also set aside enough money for offering sacrifices to appeal and appease the gods," the chief priest reminded them early.

"My son is the strongest of the men out there. That is why I should be in charge of the money," said the father of the boy who wanted to marry the most beautiful girl.

"Your son was not the only one to go, so don't assume the treasure belongs to you."

"You are all witnesses that he is attacking and insulting me again. I don't know whatever I have done to him that he won't leave me alone. He makes my life miserable. I will get back at him when the treasure arrives."

"Please, let's take it easy and respect everyone's opinion. We should all contribute our ideas and have a plan to determine how to equitably share everything. We should also plan to invest the money for the future instead of just planning a celebration."

"You are not even qualified to make any suggestions here. You have no son to give you the right to talk about choices. So stop talking and allow the men to speak," said someone. The fight continued as the villagers argued and planned a reception for the brave young men.

However, seven days into their journey and after the death of three of them, the young men suddenly found themselves in front of the entrance to the cave. They stood astounded looking at the cave. It was exactly as the hunter had described. Even though some had to pay the ultimate price, it was their dream come true. They rushed excitedly into the cave with their torches. Their mouths dropped. The cave was filled with bones, dust, and ashes. There was no gold. They saw boxes and opened them. They were filled with pebbles. The four youngsters were very upset and angry. They felt that the old hunter had sent them to the cave to die as punishment for them and the entire village. They checked everywhere but could not find any gold. They only saw boxes of pebbles and dust. Filled with anger, bitterness, and exhaustion, they started their journey back to their village. They were saddened and furious while they journeyed home. They would not even greet any passersby. Once back at the village, they headed straight to the old hunter's house, stormed in, and dragged him out.

"Why have you been so wicked? Why did you send us to the evil forest to die? Three of our friends have died a gruesome death just trying to get to the cave! When we finally arrived, there was no gold in the cave. We just saw dust and pebbles everywhere. Why did you do that to us?" They were so infuriated that they could have killed him.

The old man asked, "Did you bring anything from the cave?"

"Yes, I picked up a few pebbles to show you they are worthless." The young man that was accused of being lazy threw the bag at the old man.

The man opened it while letting the sun shine on the pebbles. It was gold. The young men were astonished. The only thing they saw inside the cave was just dusty pebbles. The young men were absolutely distraught after having returned to the village with just a few gold nuggets.

Learning From the Allegory

The young men in this story started their journey with enthusiasm and great expectations. They felt a huge sense of pride for having been chosen to represent the community on such an important expedition. Unfortunately, they did not realize the enormous sacrifice they were about to make. Their narrow minded expectation of how a gold should look like did not allow them to see the treasure before them. They returned home with what they thought were a few dusty pebbles. As they were heading back to the village with those few pebbles, they were unable to make sense of their experience. They focused their frustration on the old hunter, whom they thought would be having a good laugh at their expense. Grace is the light that helps us see the blessing of mercy and peace in the mystery of life. Much like the light of the sun that enabled the young men to see the treasure in a dusty pebble, grace allows us to see our own treasures. However, this ray of grace is not a universal light that shines everywhere. It is a light that shines on specific experiences. We have to keep our eyes open to experience this ray of grace.

When we experience suffering or someone we care about is in great distress, it is always hard to see the presence of God's grace. That is why so many people get frustrated when they hear, "Everything happens for a reason," or "It is the will of God." They may not say it, but their thought is, "Really?" That rationale falls way short from the mark. It does not always take into consideration the fact that the person suffering is in the dark, desperately trying to make sense of everything. Once people genuinely find that light, it provides comfort and peace to deal with whatever they are experiencing. They are able to find meaning in their circumstances and a place to anchor their boat floating adrift. When they proffer this meaning for themselves, it is like a beam of light in the dark.

In times of suffering, it is disheartening for us to project the universality of God's hidden intention onto each individual case. The lens of grace gives me the humility to say, "I do not know, and neither do I understand it myself." Trusting that the God of peace is there with us removes every fear from our hearts. "What then shall we say to these things? If God is for us, who can be against us? He who did not spare his own Son, but gave him up for us all—how will he not also, along with him, graciously give us all things?" (Romans 8:31). God is not finished with us. He has a plan for us. And many times, we are blind to His will for us; that is why He is offering us the grace to place our trust in Him. When Thomas asks him, "Lord, we do not know the way, please show us the way to the Father," in reply, Jesus says, "I am the way, the truth and the life" (John 11:14). This becomes an invitation to be totally dependent on Him in every situation. It is possible that we may not completely understand it. We may never know why things happen the way they do. If we face them with gentleness and calm, the experience will be different.

God uses different signs to show us that we are never alone in our suffering. The blueberries and blooming wild flower were sources of comfort to these young men. There are so many times when we are blind to the grace that God gifts us. We may feel that we see, but we really do not. It is even harder to know what we are not seeing. I lived my entire life without having to wear glasses. I always felt I could see clearly. I drove cars, rode bikes, and went around doing everything, believing that I was seeing clearly. When I went to see the optician and was tested, I read all the letters in the first line, "C U Z T R B." I also succeeded to read the second line but had to slow down: "A T B S Y D." When I got to the next line, I couldn't even attempt it. It was obvious to me that I had poor eyesight. They tried different lenses on me until they found the perfect match. The first time I used my glasses, I saw clearly and effortlessly. I shouted, "Wow!" The lens made a great difference.

The lens made me realize what poor eyesight I had. With the right lenses, we can see more clearly than we could ever imagine. Similarly, finding the right lenses could be compared to our search for meaning in life. While trying to make sense of human suffering, I started asking myself, Have I been using the wrong approach while searching for the meaning of suffering? Is it possible that we can get to understand suffering better through the lens of grace instead of theologizing about it? Do we miss the opportunity to experience grace when we focus on suffering alone? Are we missing out on grace when we are overburdened by suffering? If we are not supposed to understand suffering or make sense of it, this knowledge, or lack of it, becomes a science on its own. What if suffering wanted to be in the dark and enjoyed it? What if we were suffocating the power of love by seeking clarity to understand suffering, sickness, and disease? What if the sudden onset of suffering were deliberate in itself? Are we to create an insurance policy to prepare ourselves for when it does happen so it does not take us by surprise?

From Enthusiasts to Losers

The young men in the story saw their call as a rare privilege. They were happy to be chosen among the few to venture into the world to make a difference. They saw the gold in the wrong place. They missed the real gold and confused it with dusty pebbles. These men, in their eagerness to fetch the treasure and bring it back to the community, focused solely on the reward. They did not look at the full picture or the implications. They had a vague idea that there would be sacrifices involved. Never in their wildest dream did they think that they would experience the kind of suffering they had to endure. In the journey of life, unforeseen circumstances never come with warning labels. No one knows what is going to happen tomorrow. We may feel invincible and assume that these experiences would never happen to us. There is no immunization against pain and suffering. They are part of life. Having the abundance of grace helps us when the unexpected happens.

When we think about grace, we have a preconceived notion of what we think grace should be and look like. Sometimes, when we become proficient in a particular area of our lives, it blinds us and precludes us from seeing beyond it. Sometimes we feel that we know so much about life that there is nothing for us to learn. With a mindset like this, it is difficult to open our hearts to the possibility that there may be more than what we see. This attitude makes us narrow-minded instead of broadening our vision. The young men went to the cave and failed to see the real treasure. The secret for us lies in understanding the mystery of suffering before becoming experts in suffering.

We know so much about life and yet know so little. We consider ourselves experts on how others should live and what every other person should be doing to live a good life. This temptation to being expert consultants makes it impossible for us to listen to others. We do things because they are expected to be done in a certain way. It is the accepted norm. Therefore, it must be true. We just go with the flow or follow the crowd without taking the risk of trusting our own instinct. When the young man took the few pebbles, he must have felt in his heart that there was something to them. He was not strong enough to stand his ground to express his view or act according to his instinct. He made sure to follow instructions.

There is more than meets the eye in the story of these young men. I feel that it expresses my own internal struggle, pain, hurt, and feeling of abandonment. It reflects the danger, the fear, the poison from the snake, the anger, pride, and arrogance that kill or paralyze our hearts. It had to do with betrayal, wounds, pain, and death caused to one another. It is also the hurt we inflict on ourselves. We accept so many lies about life and suffering that they incapacitate and paralyze us, precluding us from doing what we need to for fear of shame and judgment. Those lies tell us that we are not good enough because of past mistakes, humiliations, and shame. Unfortunately, we relive them over and over, making our wounds hard to heal. We hold ourselves back and suffer the effects of that poison. We have no motivation to rid ourselves from the venom delivered to our hearts by the snake—no courage to fight for ourselves, to use our potential and the graces God bestowed upon us.

Indifference Served Cold

While these men were in the forest, living in fear, anguish, and danger of death, those in the community were fighting, politicizing, and forming committees. They were competing, planning, making laws and policies—totally ignorant of the danger these young men were enduring. Experiencing abandonment in our places of work is demoralizing. We are sometimes expected to follow procedures and protocols without regard for the human element. We theologize about suffering without any reference to the suffering and hurt experienced by the human being before us. We execute rules because a person did this or acted that way, and we fail to search for other ways. We do not even consider listening to the person in front of us because they may say something that does not fit into our script.

As I struggle with these realities, I ask myself, How many times did I fail to look at the person before me? How many times did I focus on doing what was right and expected instead of compassionately standing by the bedside of a person who carried the weight of the cross through their suffering? How many times did I judge a person because of their appearance? How many times did I judge and assumed that someone was devoid of faith because their family members judged them or others had told me so? How many times did I fail to listen to the person nailed on their cross at the hospital bed? How many times did I fail to see beauty in the brokenness of the patients before me? Did I judge their harsh words and considered them offensive instead of seeing them as a cry of anguish emanating from their heartbreak?

How many times do we take to heart what people say at the hospital? How many times do we go home brokenhearted because those in charge failed to appreciate our sacrifice? We may never realize that, much like us, those in authority are living in fear and doing what is expected. They may hide their pain and brokenness while unwittingly transferring their anxieties onto us. The physical pain we endure is negligible compared to the spiritual pain and hurt we deal with in life. Unfortunately, we tend to become enslaved by doing what is expected and can lose our identity in the process.

Receiving the gift of grace helps us in trying times so that we do not run away but dwell in peace and tranquility. We should never allow fear to make us run away from the brokenness we face. Those around us may expect us not to share our brokenness. We may choose to respect that, but their lack of understanding does not diminish our pain. Unfortunately, we tend to look away when we see suffering. We are scared to face it or witness it.

As Christians, we could easily hide under speculative theology while pontificating and legislating on what people should be doing or not doing. Like the young men in the bush, who were in anguish and despair while the villagers were at home fighting, quarreling, and speculating about who was going to get what, patients are journeying through their illnesses while their loved ones have to deal with their own feelings. We may not want to see images or hear about the tragic death of a young man whose heart was pierced by a trap. Yet parishioners, church members, and friends walk around with wounded hearts. They carry these concealed wounds and pierced hearts while bleeding inside because these wounds are to be concealed. They are hurting because of divorce, drug addiction of their family members, unemployment and afflicted by diseases. They make us uncomfortable.

We do not want to acknowledge the blood gushing out of these hearts because that is too explicit to watch. We fail to realize that these people are our brothers, sisters, friends, and members of our community. It is more comfortable to bandage and cover the wounds while they decay than provide a safe space for healing. Yes, we are afraid of asking God in tears and on bended knees to heal the pain and brokenness of our people. It is safer for us to avoid sharing in people's pain and suffering. Yet we stand by teaching them how they should carry their suffering and crosses. "Woe to you as well, experts in the law!" he replied. "You weigh men down with heavy burdens, but you yourselves will not lift a finger to lighten the burden" (Luke 11:46). We are being invited to a sacred space where suffering dwells so we may face it without shame. We ought to open ourselves up to receiving grace instead of running away from it. We are called to share in the healing grace that Jesus shares with humanity. He was not ashamed to call us His brothers. "Surely he took up our pain and bore our suffering" (Isaiah 53:4).

Part III

THE PROMISE

"Blessed is she who believed that the Lord
would fulfill His promises to her!"
(Luke 1:45)

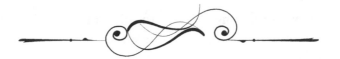

The Seal of Grace

As I grew up in a tropical country, malaria was basically a part of our everyday existence. It was never *if* but *when* you would get malaria. During my entire childhood, I never knew I had an allergy to malaria pills. One day, while at school, I felt very cold and shivery. I knew I had malaria, and I was sent home by the teacher. The ordeal that awaited me at home consisted in taking chloroquine, a malaria pill that my mother kept at home for emergencies. I thought I would get through the sickness without having to take that horrible pill that I hated. It didn't work. As I got home, I explained to my mom that I was sent home because I was sick. She placed the palm of her hand on my neck to check my temperature. She immediately gave me two pills. Being allergic to malaria medications was not considered a big deal. My mother believed that the allergy to the medication would not kill me and was rather a sign of recovery.

When I developed the allergy, no part of my body was spared. I could not sit still, stand, or lie down for thirty seconds without scratching my head or arm. In a way, the effect the allergy had on me was as if the allergic reaction were playing music with every part of my body. It struck a chord in my ear and feet, and my stomach was like a drum. I was like a puppet with strings manipulated by my allergy. The worst part was that the allergic reaction did not show on my skin, so no one could see what I was going through. My mom would determine when to stop the allergic reaction. To do this, she cracked a coconut and gave me the water to drink. That ended the itching. I was only allowed the coconut when she had determined that the fever was gone. I do not have any clinical knowledge of how coconuts stop the allergy in a child. All I knew was that drinking coconut water stopped my allergic reaction. This allergy to malaria pills reflects the conflicting reaction to suffering and the temptation when it turns overwhelming, especially when we have multiple scores to settle at the same time.

Life does pose many challenges that are multifaceted. Trials and suffering converge on us, and they terrify and disorient us. It is always traumatic and causes great anxiety for us. When these problems happen at the same time, we feel overwhelmed, helpless, and miserable. In situations such as these, when we try to solve a problem, another one erupts. While solving the most immediate one, we see a monstrous one erupting. Going through so much suffering at the same time often feels like trying to fill a bucket of water with multiple holes. If we seal one, the other ones continue to leak. Facing multiple problems is disheartening and discouraging. We are tempted to fall into despair when we face terrifying situations in life.

The Grace of Listening

A woman who had had a stroke while I was on call requested to see a chaplain, and I went to see her. She told me that her life had been crazy the past couple of weeks. She had been anxious and stressed. I sat and just listened.

"Chaplain, it was like living in hell for the last few weeks. My life is a mess right now. On the outside, everyone thinks I am fabulous—that I have money, a home, good husband, beautiful children, and fantastic friends. As a family, we just got back from a fancy vacation in the Bahamas. Unfortunately, people see what they want to see. No one wants to pay attention. No one understands what I am going through. My partial stroke is the least of my problems right now."

I thought to myself that her stroke should be her greatest concern, but didn't say anything and continued to listen.

"I don't even know where to start. Three days ago, I paid more than one thousand dollars to the vet office for Vigil. She is my dog, and she broke her hip when she jumped out of the truck. This week, I got a speeding ticket in the mail. I was picked up by a camera. I was rushing to pick my son up from a football game. I am still dealing with his coach, who thinks I am a freak. He was benching my son during most practices and games. I gave him a piece of my mind. I just got back from the hospital with my daughter, who was hospitalized. She had surgery because she broke her femur playing soccer. She had exams but was unable to take them. She will be doing confirmation soon. I have not gotten her a dress, and now she will do her confirmation on crutches.

To crown this whole disaster, my husband is cheating on me. I found out through Facebook about five days ago. Yet he came home smiling and pretended that everything was all right. I kicked him out. I told him to leave and to find another place. I could not bear to see his face after all the sacrifices I had made. He told me lies and pretended that he loved me. I am just a mess right now. I felt depleted and humiliated. So was I not good enough for him? I cannot believe that I was so blind to marry him. I am not even sure what blinded me in the first place. I still feel I should have filed for divorce at the end of our honeymoon when I realized who he was. He was clueless and did not even know what was important to me. I am very angry that he did this to me. Sorry, I am telling you all these things, but I am so upset. I have put up with him for over fifteen years. I was tempted to quit the relationship years ago like most of my friends did. I looked at my kids and thought I have to stay for the rest of the ride. I was frustrated every day. You want to know what I feel? I feel I let myself and my family down. Maybe it is my fault that all these things are happening. Maybe I allowed myself to be abused by everyone around me. I feel miserable. I don't even know where to start again.

It is deplorable that these things are happening at the same time: issues with my husband, the dog, and my daughter. My mother called and told me that they found out my dad has pancreatic cancer. All these things happening all around me? I prayed and do not even know if God still answers my prayers. The more I prayed for His help, the more He multiplied my suffering. Even my best friends, I told them my problems about my husband, and just like that, they stopped calling or texting me. They have not come to visit me at the hospital. I told my husband not to come to the hospital to see me.

As I said before, what irritates me most is that everyone felt I had the best marriage. That was such a lie!"

I sincerely listened and paid attention to this woman's pain, struggles, fears, and lamentations. What else could I have said in that situation to help her? I felt all I could do was listen to her. In all honesty, my heart went out to her. I saw the relief in her face when I sat and listened. It was a long listening session, and I was tired. It meant a lot to her, though. Having someone who can listen to us without judging when we are suffering may be an antidote for hurting. Showing compassion in that moment to someone who is going through great distress is helpful. Listening to her stories alone without saying anything to her about her crisis was like what the coconut water did for me in relieving my allergic reaction to the malaria medicine. Listening, as simple as it may sound, builds a relationship based on trust. Having someone listen to us can help us see the hidden mystery in suffering. It is only revealed to us if we pay attention to the presence of God's grace. We are drawn into a depth that goes beyond the pain and anguish we feel. The reality of physical pain may be there, but we have peace and tranquility if we feel listened to in that time of crisis and grief. This inner depth in listening is where we encounter the healing and miracle of the resurrection.

God is in us in at that moment when we feel everything is over. If we dig deep, we will find that in our suffering, God dwells in us. It is in the depths of our souls where we hear the voice of our being in its entirety. In this space, we find God's presence. "Be still, and know that I am God!" (Psalm 46:10). Beyond the anxiety, the confusion, and our fears, God is still with us. But we must listen to the voice of silence to find His presence there. I saw a quote recently which reaffirms this: "To hear the whisper of God, you must turn down the volume of the world. Find time to disconnect from everything around you and be still in His presence today. He is waiting for you to draw near." Like the prophet Elijah, God asks us to stand on the mountain to behold his presence. While we wait for Him, God reveals His presence after the fire in the gentle whisper (1 Kings 19:11–13). There is power in listening to God in silence beyond the fires, thunders, and earthquakes we face in our daily lives. God sends His angels in those moments to be with us. We will not hear the voice of God if we continue to allow the different voices around us to bombard our ears and distract us.

As the woman who had suffered the strokes spoke, I tried to find images and words that could offer her support and encouragement. I was astounded by the state of turmoil she was in. It was amazing that she felt that having a stroke was the lightest of her crosses. Within a short few days, her entire world had turned upside down and felt hopeless. I guess that was why she was scared. The doctors may not have had the time and/or the training to just sit and listen to her without judging or feeling that she was wasting their time. That was exactly what the woman needed at that moment: someone to pay attention to her, to make her aware that she mattered and that she was important. With the number of staff members that go in and out of every patient's room, there is often no time to make a connection with any individual. Everyone who enters a room is doing their job. Suffering can overwhelm us, especially when the onset is sudden and unexpected.

My first approach would have been, "Drive through, feel-good medicine," "God loves you in every situation." When we face difficulties, sometimes we just react. We do not always have the patience to wait and say a little prayer. When we react spontaneously, we tend not to wait for the grace of God to work through us. Taking a little time to pray when we are overwhelmed helps a lot. We should open up our hearts to God's grace. It is always important to let God be God and trust Him at all times. God may be inviting the patient to enter the holy of holies to experience His grace Zachariah, the father of John the Baptist. Listening to God in silence is that invitation to receive that healing grace.

Receiving the gift of grace from God is a source of comfort in suffering. This grace is more profoundly depicted in the riches of God's words found in the Bible. This invitation to grace is prevalent in Job, who exemplified the human experience of suffering at different levels. He acknowledged his limitations and gave himself permission to question God when he felt he had to. He did not allow the humiliation by his friends to prevent him from asking those crucial questions that roam in our minds. Not only was he able to articulate the reality of suffering, but he accepted it with total trust, grace, and elegance. His physical pain did not break his spirit. "But I know that my redeemer lives, and that at the end he will stand on the earth" (Job 19:25). Another example will be the thorn in Paul's flesh that tormented him. He was in the hands of physicians who did all they could to help him. He prayed about it over and over again and asked God that he would remove it, but nothing happened. It was uncomfortable for Saint Paul as a minister of God to know that God healed others and did not grant his request of healing for himself. He was encumbered in doing God's work of spreading the good news by this terrible pain in his flesh. He prayed earnestly to God to remove that cross. God replied to him, "My grace is sufficient for you, for my power is made perfect in weakness" (2 Corinthians 12:9). God did not physically appear to him to bring him words of comfort in his affliction. He must have communicated with Paul through different means: a whisper, dream, birds, inner voice, sky, or even through a stranger. Paul really listened to hear what God was saying to him.

The Grace of Praying

Hospital experiences could be a valuable time that draws us closer to God. Facing multiple crises at the same time is crushing. We have to call on the Lord in our moment of despair and believe He will answer us. "Cast all your cares on the Lord and He will sustain you" (Psalm 55:22). When everything else around us has failed, we have to know that God never fails, and He will never give up on us. We have to cry out to him for help when we are in anguish. "Lord, let your ear be attentive to the prayer of this your servant and to the prayer of your servants who delight in revering your name" (Nehemiah 1:11). "I love the Lord, for he heard my voice; he heard my cry for mercy" (Psalm 116:1).

I have come to believe there is power in prayer. Many testimonies show what God has done for those who put their trust in Him. We are not any different. "Then they cried to the Lord in their trouble, and He saved them from their distress" (Psalms 107:3). God is

God, and He will always stand by us in times of difficulty. It is our responsibility to cry out to Him when we are in pain and scared. We cannot keep quiet, not pray, and expect things to happen. We pray and then trust in God that His will be done in our lives. Jesus asked Saint Peter to go to him by walking on water. Peter was able to do that as long as his focus was on the Lord. "But when he saw the wind, he was afraid, and beginning to sink, cried out, 'Lord, save me!'" (Matthew 14:30). As we experience our own fear, pain, and sickness, it is important to cry out to God and say, "Lord, save me!" He is there to save us in times of need. Things may not always work the way we expect. We enjoy greater comfort and peace within ourselves through His grace.

One of the ways in which we know God is with us is when we experience His caring presence in prayer. When we cry out to God in pain and agony, God is not in the distance. He comes to sit and is with us at that moment. It is only in prayer that we connect with God's presence and experience Him being with us. Without praying and asking, how can we know that He is there to answer us? The psalmist says, "In my distress I called to the Lord; I cried to my God for help. From his temple he heard my voice; my cry came before him, into his ears" (Psalm 18:6). This is a personal testimony of the writer of this psalm. In our own individual ways, God answers whenever we cry out to Him. When you pray, you also have to mean it. Mean what you say and name that about which you pray. It is God's job to answer us. Prayer comes from our heart and not only the formal prayers.

Sarah, the wife of Abraham, prayed for years and could not conceive a child of her own. She had to let Abraham sleep with the slave girl Hagar for Abraham to have a son. Hagar gave birth to Ishmael. "But in God's own time, Isaac was born" (Genesis 17). The life of Samuel, Samson, David, Ruth and Naomi. all bear witness to God's unexplainable plan. He may appear silent to us in times of suffering, but His silence speaks volumes. We hear the story of Elizabeth and the birth of John the Baptist. Mary and all the other miracles Jesus and the disciples did in the New Testament are testimonies of God's undying love and kindness to us. He does not abandon us in times of need, and nothing is impossible for Him. He has the final word. Whatever doors He opens, no one can close; and whatever doors He closes, no one can open (Isaiah 22:22). May God open the doors to His grace daily and put a smile on your face. May no sickness or illness ever disturb the walls of your house. May He heal every cell therein and seal up and bandage every wound in you. May He uproot everything that is not of Him. For those who are barren, may you conceive and carry your child to delivery without any complication in the womb again! May God fill your heart with joy and peace and let His face shine on you!

Give the Gift of Your Presence

Growing up in Nigeria, I still remember a song we heard on the radio during the '80s by William Onyeabor: "When the going is smooth and good, many, many people will be your friend…But when the going becomes tough, many of your friends will run away." This is true in life. There will be very few people who will stick by us when things go awry. The reality in life is that we will have more followers on Facebook, Instagram, Twitter, or any other social media when things are going well than in times of need. When we are in trouble, so many of those who "loved" our posts will abandon us. Some may not have the strength to bear the cross with us. We all deal with suffering in different ways. People try to avoid suffering and pain. It is not necessarily that they do not care. They are afraid. They do not want to talk about sickness. To the one hurting, it almost feels like their message is, "It is your problem. Deal with it."

The woman who had suffered a minor stroke was hurting because her close friends were not there for her. After she confided in them about her marriage crisis, they abandoned her. They ran to their safe zone and did not want to be burdened by her. When they heard she was admitted to the hospital, they did not show up. Whereas I understand that fear might have prevented them from visiting her, my intention is not to trivialize the situation. The point is that this could happen to anyone of us at any given time. Even our friends may one day avoid us for fear of doing or saying the wrong things in the face of suffering. At the Garden of Gethsemane, Jesus felt this terrible loneliness when He was abandoned by the disciples, those He healed, fed, and performed miracles for. So He told His disciples, "You will leave me all alone. Yet I am not alone, for my Father is with me" (John 16:32).

Hospital experiences can be tremendously lonely. We fear abandonment and loneliness during those times when we need companionship the most. Having the support and presence of friends and family at the hospital will always be cherished. Conversely, being too present or overstaying could also be detrimental to patients as it does not allow them enough rest. When friends see us sick, they get scared of seeing us in those conditions. Many patients look differently when sick, especially without makeup, a proper shower, and dressed in the hospital gown. Many friends and family members are distressed when visiting sick patients. They struggle to find the right things to say, things that are not insensitive but that show their compassion and care in times of suffering. I wish there was a comprehensive manual that we could use with all the right words for hospital patients.

The gifts of presence and hospital visits come from the heart. That is where the seat of grace dwells. We do not have to say anything. Love is what matters most. Sometimes our friends may say something unexpected. They may feel they have to say something to show they care. They feel compelled to tell us things that will brighten our day and help us cope with recovery. Unfortunately, some of the things people say may be unintentionally misguided. They come out of ignorance of how to deal with suffering and sickness. We do not want to say anything wrong while tending to the sick. There are times, however, when people say things assuming that they will help the patient, but they do not. It would have been better for them to have kept quiet. Some of the things we frequently hear at the hospital—"God has His reasons," for example—hurt more than help as the patient tries to process what the reason could be.

We hear all the wonderful things God has done, and we believe He will be there for us to heal us in times of sickness. Times do come when we are frightened and panic when facing problems and temptations. Sometimes we are terrified because the answer to our prayers for healing are delayed or do not come at all. This creates doubt in our minds about God's providence and presence. Gideon laid his heart to God:

> "Pardon me, my Lord," Gideon replied, "but if the Lord is with us, why has all this happened to us? Where are all his wonders that our ancestors told us about when they said, 'Did not the Lord bring us up out of Egypt?' But now the Lord has abandoned us and given us to the hand of Midian." (Judges 6:13)

Those times when we feel alone and abandoned by friends or family, we have to know that we are never alone. God stands with us through the nurses and staff who enter the room to perform one job or another. Through them, God's promises are being fulfilled because he has so many ways to show us He cares. He may not manifest Himself in a physical form, but if we open our eyes, we can see Him through all those He is using to perform healing miracles in our lives. This will help us to understand His promise, "When you go through deep waters, I will be with you" (Isaiah 43:2). No matter the suffering, we all share in the cross of Christ. Others share in the same suffering with us. Saint Paul united his suffering with Christ's and the whole church. "Now I rejoice in what I am suffering for you, and I fill up in my flesh what is still lacking in regard to Christ's afflictions, for the sake of his body, which is the Church" (Colossians 1:24).

The Inestimable Gift of Patience

In all fairness, life is not fair. Things do not always turn out the way we want, and patience is not one of those virtues that flows easily for so many of us. As humans, we are not always patient. We want things done and done fast. We want immediate answers and results. We want to know and know fast. Waiting could be a frustrating experience at the hospital. It is worse when we do not have answers or have the end in sight. Waiting is filled with uncertainty.

It is stressful. It is never easy to plan and have a strategy in times of uncertainty. We are always encouraged to be patient and wait. Who among us is comfortable waiting for anything? I am not sure I am among them. Like the woman who had the stroke, when we face multiple setbacks at the same time, which one of them could wait and be taken care of later? Honestly, it is very difficult to be patient and wait, not reacting to situations. It is something that we easily talk about but is very hard to do. Waiting is a great grace that is always helpful in every situation. Going the extra mile and waiting may be the greatest help to our millions of problems. The psalmist invites us, "Wait for the Lord; be strong and take heart and wait for the Lord" (Psalm 27:14). We need to be strong to wait because we feel that waiting is an act of weakness. Clearly, it is an act of strength to wait patiently for anything as we pray about it.

Waiting silently for God does not mean being passive or nonchalant. It means opening our eyes to take in more details and read in between the lines of things we take for granted. It is an invitation for a deeper relationship with the things before us. In times of difficulty, we should not allow ourselves to be distracted by minutia. Sometimes there is a hidden abundance of grace being revealed. This grace takes time to unfold. We have to pray, have faith, and wait. There is a depth to our being that allows us to see grace if we wait. This is the indwelling of the Holy Spirit that is already in us. We need to allow this grace to work in us.

Waiting could test our patience and push us to the limit. It could also be stressful when we focus our thoughts on what people may or may not be saying to us. At the hospital, we have no control of things around us, and we have to learn to be patient. The way in which we wait when we wait is very important. Do we wait in agitation and become flustered? Do we wait, hoping for the best? Knowing God is there with us gives us hope that we are not abandoned. That is the grace that is a source of comfort. Feeling God's presence helps us wait. We do not depend on the outcome to be at peace. We have peace and grace while we wait in hope. The grace of waiting becomes like the example I gave of my mother and the malaria pills. She deliberately waited to make sure the malaria was gone before giving me the coconut water to stop my allergic reaction to the malaria pill. Her priority was making sure I would fully recover. She was able to watch me suffer the allergic reaction only because she knew that malaria was worse.

Suffering is not something easy to grasp. I do not think anyone enjoys it. It would be good to live in a world where there was no sickness, disease, accident, mental illness, suicide, war, greed, hunger, betrayal, or any form of evil. The truth is that such world does not exist. Each of us faces temptation on a daily basis. Sometimes temptation is very enticing and treacherous, other times chronic and difficult to overcome. How do we react to temptation? What do we do to overcome it? What can we do to find grace in our vulnerability?

Saint Theresa of Avila said, "Let nothing disturb you: Nothing frighten you. All things are passing. God never changes. Patience obtains all things. Nothing is wanting to him who possesses God. God alone suffices." Being hospitalized is one thing; how we deal with our condition is another. The unspoken word, the faces of those who enter our rooms, the pain we go through, and the uncertainty after discharge are all interwoven experiences. This experience is how we open the doors for grace to flow. If we find God in the darkest moments of our lives, we have found peace. This inner peace removes every anxiety and stress from us.

The story of the woman who had a stroke is an example of what we go through when suffering comes in a multifaceted way. It is disorienting. We are only able to deal with it by the grace of God. This lady's family crisis was more important to her than having had a stroke or a biopsy. I had a long talk with her that day. When I entered her room another day to check on her, her face lit up. "Thank you, Chaplain, for coming again. What you did for me yesterday meant a lot. You were my saving grace. I felt invisible and that no one was really interested in me. I felt I was just a research specimen because I had had stroke. All those who walked into my room saw me as a patient with a stroke. They only wanted to talk about the disease, and I felt I was not a person. You were a breath of fresh air. You made me feel precious. That changed everything for me. I was with my husband today, and he left to get lunch. The fear I had of him cheating on me vanished. His sister had sent him the contact for an eighth-grade friend of theirs when she had run into her. She acknowledged there was nothing fishy about the relationship." I was happy that it all ended well. If we do not listen to ourselves, to God, others around us, we may continue to react. It is the grace of God that heals and strengthens us. We must drink from the fountain of that grace the same way I had to drink the coconut water to stop my allergic-reaction dance.

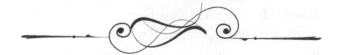

Complaining Creates Tension

We unknowingly tend to complain on our way to glory. Though the journey of life is tough, it is also filled with moments of laughter and joy. Complaining casts shadows on the graces that dwell in suffering and sickness. It beclouds those moments of grace that provide us with a small window of opportunity to take a deep breath before continuing. If we complain and whine, our journey becomes harder, longer, and more difficult. Could you imagine how long the journey to the top of the mountain would be if all we did was complain about how rough the road was? If we kept talking about our fear of coming face-to-face with a bear or a poisonous snake, we would certainly change the entire dynamic of the journey. That does not mean that we should not express our emotions or speak out against injustice. If complaining does not help us make changes, how is that helpful? Expressing our concern could be grace-filled if we do it in the spirit of justice, and we do not become consumed by it.

Suffering and struggle carry hidden glory. Although suffering does not make sense to us, there is glory in it. Complaining closes the door for us to experience grace. Life is tough, but it is all about perspective. If we choose to whine and complain, we can do that, or we could choose to see the beauty being revealed in every cross we bear. We all make sacrifices during our journey. Complaining about a situation does not help us move along. As we climbed to the mountaintop, the road was very difficult, rough, and riddled with slippery rocks. However, all of us, including the staff and students, continued to focus on the peak of the mountain, and we found the motivation to keep going. That became the drive that helped us cope with any temporary discomfort. Complaining about things does not change anything but aggravates the situation and creates more tension.

Not everyone received the gift to never complain as some saints did. In my case, whenever I am happy, my face bursts with joy. If I am sad, that sadness shows. If I taste a delicious dish, I exclaim, "Wow! That is wonderful." I really can't hide it if I don't like it. I have heard myself say, "This is different." Even if I don't say anything, my face would show it. If I am sick, everyone would definitely know. I cannot imagine myself keeping quiet if I was in pain.

Complaining is something that we often do instinctively and naturally. It is important to keep this attitude in check as it hurts us more than it helps. Whining about a situation does not necessarily translate into finding a solution. I often complained about those in authority, be it government, church leaders, or private organizations. I often feel that employees working at bureaucratic offices become blind and deaf to the reality and needs of others. Those in authority often want to see what they want to see and close their eyes to other possibilities.

It is worrisome to see the ineptitude of many in leadership around the world. While those in positions of power are the ones who set the course for others, many of them are the primary cause of poverty. In many countries, leaders squander the economic and human resources of the very communities they were elected to lead and protect. I got used to lamenting and complaining about them, about what they were doing wrong, about what they should have been doing, and about how bad they were. The more I watched the daily news, read the news, or talked about them, the more disappointed, disheartened, and hopeless I became. One day I told myself I had had enough, and I had peace.

As I rattled off and complained about how unjust and unfair most of those in authority were, I neglected to notice the quiet, selfless leaders of our world. It is not only about the office. It is our ability to use the office to serve humanity. Grace allowed me to see that complaining about those in authority and discussing how bad things looked caused unnecessary and unproductive stress. Little did I know that watching the news was detrimental to my spiritual life. Even though I could potentially come up with a solution in my head, I could not affect change alone. That was when I started to pray more for those in authority instead of complaining about them. By the grace of God, I was able to see their limitations and that they need God's grace more than anyone. We generally hold them to very high standards.

Through the story of the people of Israel, we can see how they experienced grace in their suffering and how they transformed those experiences even as they trusted God to save them. We clearly understand that our suffering is not punishment because of sin. The social ills we go through are a consequence of human greed and selfishness. God is not here to inflict pain and suffering on humanity. He was never desensitized to the suffering of people. If we look at the Israelites, God was there with them, although the realization of God's presence took a while. He stood with them when they suffered. He was never a God sheltered in heaven and all its beauty. God was always part of their journey and their story. This is clearly seen in the various ways He manifested His caring presence for them in their journey from Egypt to the Promised Land. Learning from their story will help us find meaning in our own suffering.

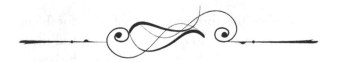

The Grandeur of Grace

Every culture has its story to show the infinite goodness of God, or of a supreme being, that portrays the limits of human ability and resources. So many stories are told to offer meaning in times of suffering. These stories describe in amazing ways the almightiness of God through His intervention in human existence. Throughout the ages, there have been folk stories, fables, myths, and parables attempting to satisfy our human hunger to explain this mystery. I marvel at the wisdom and sacredness of these stories and their attempt to open our eyes to experience beauty and grace even in our darkest times. These stories become resurrection experiences that shed light on grace and reconnects us with God's Word.

The Reconnection to the Word

The Israelites' journey from slavery in Egypt to the Promised Land is one of the greatest stories ever written to express the reality of suffering. This story presented the human quality of the Israelites— their fears, doubts, anger, hunger, sickness, death, and what they went through to fulfil this promise. The Israelites acknowledged that God was part of their journey. They were led by Moses through the desert and suffered hardship, brutal pestilence, harsh weather, famine, fear, and uncertainty. They journeyed in these conditions clinging to the hope of the Promised Land: a land flowing with milk and honey. They taught their children that their success story was not a right but a gift from God, who was their provider and healer. It was an invitation to be grateful for their story and not to be ashamed.

> Remember the former things of old, for I am
> God, and there is no other; I am God, and there
> is none like me, declaring the end from the begin-
> ning, and from ancient times things that are not
> yet done, saying, "My counsel shall stand, and I
> will do all my pleasure." (Isaiah 46:9–10)

Hence, they recalled the wonderful things God did, how He used nature to fight for their ancestors. They reminded their children that they were God's chosen people. They taught them that despite the hardship they may have experienced, God will always give them victory if they hold on to Him to the end. For instance, the Bible recorded that one of their leaders, Joshua, prayed that the sun should stand still. The sun stopped in the middle of the sky and delayed going down about a full day. They were victorious in battle because of Joshua (Joshua 10:12–14). The testimony of the Israelites is a record of resilience, the power of hope in times of hopelessness, and the gift of grace in their darkest moments.

The pain we face daily is clearly mirrored after the Israelites' exodus to the Promised Land. It is very important to always remember that the desert is not a living place. It is barren and empty, a place where nothing grows. When the people of Israel left Egypt, they left with the hope of getting to the Promised Land quickly. The desert was a transitional place for their journey. It was a temporal experience as they journeyed to their destination. Yet it took them forty years in the desert to get to the Promised Land.

Getting to the Promised Land was possible only because the Israelites reconnected with their roots and faith. They recalled what God did for their ancestors: He was there in the desert with them. He was there to open their eyes to see water on the rock, the manna, quail; and when bitten by snakes, they looked at the molded snake to live. They moved with uncertainty, yet they trusted the promises God had made through Moses and other leaders. The Israelites remembered their history, their story, and their roots. They knew God would journey with them till the end because He was there for their ancestors. Those stories reignited their energy to continue their journey. This is what faith is all about. Hope in our faith is what keeps us going.

The Attainment of Illumination

Like the Israelites, the stories and testimonies of the past help to build up our faith. We get to that level in which we experience tremendous peace in the face of adversity. Whenever we feel we are journeying through the desert, alone, abandoned and desperate, we must remember that God walks by our side. Anytime we go through difficult situations, He is there to help us. The same way He provided for the people of Israel, He will provide for us. As He guided and protected them until they got to the Promised Land, He will protect us. The people of Israel did not remain in the desert forever, and our difficulties also have expiration dates. The only thing that is required of us is to trust God's providence.

We are always saddened and fearful as we go through life's desert. It breaks and humiliates us and makes us do bizarre things. These desert experiences are not the end of the story; they are only the beginning. The fullness of the story is that in the desert, God was with His people. The same God who was there with the Israelites when they experienced their darkest moment in history is our companion in everyday life. When they cried out to Him, He answered them. They listened to Him speak through Moses and the prophets. They watched and waited to see the signs that made them realize his presence. They persevered in their prayers and never gave up hope because of the faith they had in God for what He had done and what they believed He would do. We have to wait, watch, and listen to know the answers to our cry and prayers so we do not hope or wait in vain. He journeys with us through those muddy and rocky roads. He is not a God who stays in the distance to watch us go through the heat alone. He is our companion.

In the face of suffering, how do we know that God cares? How do we feel He is present when all our senses tell us differently? The impact of a tragedy is so staggering that our senses become paralyzed and drained. Our physical and emotional energy is gone, and we are not able to see, feel, touch, or hear anything. Can you imagine receiving a devastating call while at a party? No matter how delicious the food, in the face of tragedy, it would mean nothing.

One day, I went to see a patient who radiated such joy with a lovely smile. I told her, "With this face, I bet the nurses will frequent your room just to see your smile." Her face beamed and glowed with such yearning and glory that you couldn't but adore her. She replied, "Thanks. I came to the hospital yesterday. I started having a headache last week and had to take some painkillers. Yesterday, I felt weird and nauseous, so I decided to see my family doctor. He sent me here for an MRI. This morning, they just told me that I have an inoperable brain tumor that is aggressively spreading. I have a few weeks or months to live. I allowed them to leave my room. I closed my eyes and screamed. I was concerned because of my daughters. I had an unbelievable sense of peace about it. I felt God's grace in my heart. It was not a coincidence that the scripture I read yesterday, the morning before going to the hospital, was Psalm 119: 48:

> I revered your commandments, which I love, and I will meditate on your statues. Remember your word to your servant, in which you have made me hope. This is my comfort in my distress, that your promise gives me life. The arrogant utterly deride me, but I do not turn away from your law. When I think of your ordinances from old, I take comfort, O Lord. (Psalm 119:48–52)

"I believe that God is with me and will be with me through it all."

I stood in awe of her. With this devastating news, how could she still be in good spirits, show such expressions of love and grace? How is this possible? The jolly spirit with which I had entered her room instantly disappeared. I was curious and asked her, "How did you find peace and grace so quickly after being delivered such dire news?" Her answer was surprising: "The psalm that morning was God's personal message to me, letting me know that He is with me. I know that this suffering is real, but He opened my eyes to know that He is with me. I felt alive in Him with those words, and they gave me life."

God shows us in different ways His ever-abiding and caring presence. These moments of illumination are neither reproducible nor explainable. Witnessing God's abundant grace and miracles builds a solid faith for us. They help shape our personal faith, even when we are not able to communicate what we witnessed. That healing testimony is our own spiritual DNA. This personal and internal experience of God is what gives meaning to our suffering. That tiny voice is what sparks up that inner hope and builds the connection we need to forge on because God is with us. This healing is not necessarily physical or automatic. Miracles do happen. Another way to heal is by finding purpose and meaning in those awkward moments. It is having the wealth of grace to process things into purposefulness instead of accepting them as powerless or limiting our potential. We change our narrative by overcoming our predicaments and dispelling darkness and influencing others even at our weakest.

To carry our cross alone is always hard no matter the shape or size. Jesus journeys with the weak and the broken. He is there with them and not the strong and mighty. When Jesus becomes our companion on the journey, the pain and the burden of the load becomes lighter. When we have a stronger friend to accompany us on our journey, the weight becomes lighter as they help. Jesus is someone who can comfortably carry it on our behalf and make us walk with Him. He is a companion that tells us stories as we walk along the road with Him on our journey. Those companions are our friend Jesus and our mother Mary. We do not feel the heat of the sun when we have a loved one and a friend as our companion. The journey does not even seem long when we are laughing, smiling, and enjoying it. If we journey with someone we don't like, we feel lonely, terrified, and the distance becomes glaringly long.

The Courage to Hope

Experiences of failure and shame could be detrimental to our hope. They could make us feel that hoping is a waste of time. It is an illusion to hope because it hurts more when we fail to achieve what we had hoped. Hence, it would be better not to try, fail, and go through the pain of humiliation. As we attempt to explore new options in hope of success, it is easier to bear the pain of failure alone. There is no certainty in hope. There is no need to expect anything or waste one's time hoping because we may end up disappointed. What is certain, though, is what we do have and not what we hope for. *That* is uncertain and unpredictable. At times, we get what we hope for, but most times, heartbreak ensues. So in order not to feel disappointed, it is better not to hope. Fight for what you believe and live for today and forget about putting your trust in the hope of tomorrow. Hence, you will not experience the pain of hoping for a brighter and better future. Unfortunately, this attitude leads to despair not resiliency.

I could not think of much at that moment but remembered that when all else fails, God is there. Clinging to Him in difficult times brings comfort and consolation. It pulls us away from despair. If I had a few days to live, what would I do? For sure, I would be devastated; and honestly, I would probably not know what to do next. It would hurt badly, to put it mildly. That is why I would only ask God for grace at that time of darkness. "The Lord will surely comfort Zion and will look with compassion on all her ruins… Joy and gladness will be found in her, thanksgiving and the sound of singing" (Isaiah 51:3). God is my only hope in time of darkness. Without this hope in Him, I am dead.

God's ways are not our ways, and His understanding is not ours. I don't know and neither do I understand why things happen the way they do. But believing that God is there with me in every moment offers me peace of mind. Like a child left alone in the house, the voice of the mom is a source of comfort. I could only find comfort in God's arms. He is there with me in many inexplicable ways. He made me experience His presence even in darkness.

> Why do you complain, Jacob? Why do you say,
> Israel, my way is hidden from the Lord; my cause
> is disregarded by my God? Do you not know?

Have you not heard? The Lord is the everlasting God, the creator of the ends of the earth. He will not grow tired or weary, and his understanding no one can fathom. He gives strength to the weary and increases the power of the weak. (Isaiah 40:27–29)

The hope that is anchored in God has an abundance of grace that flows with it. God reveals the mystery of His presence even in the worst catastrophes. This blessing is a revelation that can only be contemplated through the eyes of innocence. It is not about what we see or feel. It is the richness of the goodness of the Lord as He pours it abundantly on us. This is what the Samaritan woman at the well experienced. She found the fountain that never runs dry in Jesus. She runs to her town to be the first evangelist: "I have found someone who told me everything" (John 4:4–26). It is the inner awareness of the presence of God and His ability to help us in time of need that pulls us through in times of crisis and difficulty.

God's greatness is unfathomable, and His abiding presence is forevermore. We are invited to share in this infinite bliss of His goodness. Hope opens the door for us to tap into it. We have to go beyond the human logic and calculations to see that God could do things in his own way. It enables us to hear that while we cry, God cries with us. He shares in our brokenness. "Do I take pleasure in the death of the wicked? Declares the sovereign Lord. Rather, am I not pleased when they turn from their ways and live?" (Ezekiel 18:23).

The mystery of grace is to open our hearts to find God's revelation in times of suffering. What is God saying to us when we are broken in the dark? What is being revealed to us in that sacred moment when we are without hope? It is only in the encounter with the Divine Master where we can find the inner strength to cope in times of great distress. Only God can teach and reveal the interconnectedness between the pain, fear, confusion, and suffering that we experience and the grace dwelling therein. Grace is inseparable from suffering and pain. They are intertwined. It is in openness where grace finds meaning in the face of meaninglessness.

Christian hope defies logic and expectation. The widow at Zarephath gave up hope even while obeying the words of the Prophet Elijah. "As surely as the Lord your God lives," she replied, "I don't have any bread—only a handful of flour in a jar and a little olive oil in a jug. I am gathering a few sticks to take home and make a meal for myself and my son, that we may eat it—and die." Elijah said to her, "Don't be afraid. Go home and do as you have said." She went away and did as Elijah had told her" (1 Kings 17:7–16). As she obeyed the words of the prophet, the jar of oil flowed in abundance. God was there with her. The surpassing goodness of God flows into our hearts to bring us comfort. This hope is always there even when we don't see it. This hope is what God revealed to us and continuously reveals to us so we are drawn to His generous abundance. This is an opportunity to relive and rewrite our story. This is what happened to the Israelites. They learned from their mistakes and tried to live again. There are many ways God has shown us that grace of His presence to be hopeful in the midst of suffering. He sends us messages of comfort even through dreams.

Signs Rekindle Our Hope

While searching for answers filled with hopelessness, God often shows us His enduring presence through signs. We all have our own individual experience of the signs that emerge when we are battling to find answers. We watch those signs in disbelief and awe! We may not be able to name them and may call them miracles, coincidences, accidents, magic, or whatever, but they are real to us. Those moments of grace are moments of healing. We are left speechless. The experience is so real that even when people think we are deluded, we know what an overpowering and transforming experience we have had. Nothing anyone can say will ever erase those signs, images, or experiences.

Therefore, it is never because we are not good enough that things do not happen exactly the way we want, when we want, and how we want. At times, trusting our dependable God is all we can do. Knowing the immensity of His love strengthens our heart because, as in Song of Songs, "He has brought me to the banquet hall, and his banner over is love" (Song of Songs 2:4). This knowledge of His ever-abiding presence keeps us afloat at sea during times of stormy waters. Without that grace, we are not stable. We live in fear and despair. God promises, "Can a mother forget the baby at her breast and have no compassion on the child she has borne? Though she may forget, I will not forget you" (Isaiah 49:15). This implies that God has not forgotten us, and neither has He neglected us. When we are terrified, Jesus whispers to us, "Take courage! It is I. Don't be afraid" (Matthew 14:27).

These signs strengthen us in our journey and build that hope that motivates us to the end. These personal experiences validate the reality of God's caring presence for us. Those signs tend to give us hope and speak to our need. They help us realize there is light at the end of the tunnel. Like when Noah saw the rainbow, it was a sign of great hope for him and those with him. It was a sign that God will never allow the universe to be destroyed by floods again. God speaks to every individual in a particular way even in the midst of pain and anguish. But we must wait to see those signs. We must pay attention so we do not miss the sign or take it for granted.

I sent a text message to my friend in an attempt to share with her how we encounter God in the emptiness of silence. His presence heals us far more than what we have been taught or what we thought were right theological answers. Her testimony and our chat make this crystal clear. I am copying the text as is and without edits:

> In [this] silence we are told we hear God, but it's not always so. I know when I was so lost and heartbroken, I cried and cried, and cried over many, many months. Then, once, as I was sitting quietly with my eyes closed, Jesus came to me. I saw it in my mind and he wrapped his arms around me and I had my head on his chest. He held me so tight as I cried. It brings tears to my eyes when I think of it. I miss [doing] that with my dad, my mom and my brother so very much, we always hugged.

Then I responded by saying, "You see how that speaks to your heart. Your personal experience of Jesus wrapping His arms around you is a sign that God cares for us always. That's your personal experience of who God is, and it is what gives meaning to our life. That is more important than anything anyone could teach us."

> Yes, but it took so long for me to begin to heal. My brother was a profound loss to me. I was so angry at God. I waited for my brother to be revived [sic]. I was certain of it and believed it. That's where I went wrong. My belief was too great. When it didn't happen, I was shattered. It was a beautiful moment I will remember always. It felt so good to have him hold me.

"What healed you was not something someone told you. It was encountering Jesus in that space by yourself and that comfort [of knowing] that you are safe. That's what is great about it."

> Yes, on the way up to my brother's funeral, I saw not one but three rainbows. When I stopped at the last light there was the last rainbow. A woman pulled up alongside of me. She rolled her window down and said, "Look at that rainbow. It's a gift from God and it's going to be all right. I didn't know her. I took a photo of the rainbows and [for] the last one, there was an image in it; and the telephone pole looks like a cross. The rainbow, the woman and the poles that looked like the cross…It was a sign."

What signs are there for us to realize that God is with us in every situation? I have had moments in my own life when, through little signs, I feel God's presence with me. I may not be able to explain it well to someone else. Those are things that keep the presence of God alive in us because He is real to us. God's caring presence is also substantial in the different signs He shows us individually. These signs can be the presence of a rare bird when it is absolutely unexpected. It may be through water, things in nature, a plant, song, animal, or different objects. There are times God sends angels in the form of humans to come be with us. Those little signs are God's manifestations of how much He cares for us. He is a God, who is there with us even in the dirt and mud, and He will not abandon us.

There are times when God's compassionate presence is made real through dreams. Each one of us may still remember a few of those dreams throughout our lives. They, at times, serve as the connection to finding the answer to who we are. They help in providing meaning and relevance as we grapple for answers in our search for sustenance in dark times. Dreams do address and speak to our needs. They help in many ways by providing unimaginable answers to our life's situation.

Through my own dreams, I have encountered God's abiding presence that in my brokenness, there is the assurance that He cares. Dreams could become a means to encountering God's presence. The Bible has so many dream testimonies of God revealing His plan to His children to offer them support and encouragement in difficult times. Joseph dreamed and waited for years in anticipation and uncertainty for the fulfilment of those dreams. Hope saves us from despair, and hope has its foundation on expectation. I am sure many of us must have had a dream. Our ability to understand the implication of those dreams help fulfill our quest for answers too. Such experiences speak to the heart of our being and enable us to experience God's presence in our brokenness.

Think of your own life. How many times have we had a dream that we felt was real? How often do we receive answers, hope, or strength to mind-boggling questions through our dreams? When our dreams add meaning to our everyday life and existence, they become an encounter with God. Dreams are our stories, our life, and part of our entire being. When we dream, it is not just a dream; it is a meaningful message that could serve a useful purpose. Sometimes we find consolation, strength, significance in those messages, and we realize that they are God's gift of grace to us. Our God stands with us, and we are important to Him. "My beloved is mine and I am his; he browses among the lilies" (Song of Songs 2:16). Through these experiences of the Israelites, we see that in their agonizing suffering, they were determined to change their conditions and not accept helplessness. They did that by appreciating the gift of God and sharing in the story of their redemption.

Part IV

THE TRANSFORMATION

"I have heard your prayers and seen your
tears; I will heal you" (2 Kings 20:5).

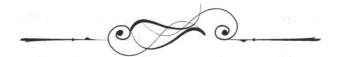

Restoration Is Indispensable

Dancing in the rain! Playing in the moonlight! Listening to stories and singing while the corn exploded by the fire! Chasing fireflies and lizards—I miss all of that so much. I miss those holy childhood moments. I miss the fun, the little lies, the foolishness, the stubbornness, the hiding games, the mischievousness, and the innocence. It was fun. It was messy, dirty, playful, frightful, sacred, and graceful. I would love to have that back, but I can't. That grace was the fountain of my being. How I wish those waters of abundant joy could be reclaimed. I wish I could push off the burden of fear and shame grown-ups experience to behold the beauty and innocence of being a child again. There was delight, freshness, and excitement in being a child. I know I can't get that childlike life back, but I could live in freedom, joy, peace, and grace like a child. As we enjoyed and played with antlions during my childhood, their steps and backward movements serve as a reminder that we should appreciate the gift of yesterday as we live today. We should not postpone living today as we prepare for tomorrow. It was a lesson in my dialect, *onye ma echi*, which translated means, "No one knows tomorrow." We also say *echi di ime*, which means, "Tomorrow is pregnant, and no one knows the child tomorrow will give birth to." Tomorrow is filled with uncertainty. We must live fully today to prepare for the future.

Growing up in Nigeria, we used to play with little creatures in the mud: ants, antlions, crickets, butterflies, caterpillars, and spiders. I still remember the song we sang for the ant lions as we lay in the mud, "Kpukpu kpo ogene kpuo ogene kpuo ogene ge. Onye na akpo ogene? Kpo ogene, kpuo ogenege. Ewu na-akpo ogene, kpo ogene, kpo ogene ge. Kpuu kpuu, kpo ogene, kpo ogenege." While we had fun, I never paid attention to the meaning of what we sang. It turns out that we were pretending to knock to invite the ant lion to come out and play with us, and the ant lions would respond, "Who is knocking?" We would pretend different animals like goats, chickens, and cows were inviting the ant lions to come out to play.

The ant lions were little insects that dug tiny holes in the soft sand. They walked backward and, while doing that, burrowed in the ground to bring out some soft sand to the surface. Each of them lived in their individual dugouts alone. As kids, we went around searching for signs of their holes. When we found them, we lay on the ground, sang, and tapped our hands on the ground following the rhythm of the music until they came out. It was absolutely terrific to watch the backward movement of this creature as it burrowed in the ground trying to come out. We had fun and got our clothes very dirty. We were never ashamed of being dirty because we were playing. Being dirty or naked was a problem for grown-ups. For us, having fun and running around in mud with other kids was sheer bliss. The mess and dirt were part of us, and we loved and enjoyed every bit of it.

Today, as I woke up to write this reflection, the song in my mind was "Kpuu kpuu kpo ogene" for ant lions and humanity. I know I can't find that insect where I live right now, and I cannot go back to lie on the mud to play with the ant lions. The song was a way to recall the grace and beauty of the messy world we live in. It is the sacredness of each and every one of us joining in play. It is the understanding that we are all part of the imperfection and the muckiness as we enjoy the blessings of our world. *Kpuu kpuu* was a voice to us all, a daily reminder that we should not dwell in the ugliness without grace. It was a call to open ourselves up to the reality of pain, joy, and suffering. We are called to approach it somewhat playfully so we are not chocked up by the ugliness. We are living in a far-from-perfect world, and we are all part of it. It is an invitation for each and every one of us to be part of that game again.

Like the ant lions that burrow in the earth to build their safe and comfortable space in loneliness, we too may have all the comforts of life and still face woes. Without hearing the sound of the invitation to play, we fail to recognize that the fun of life lies in the beauty of living. This invitation for the ant lion to come out from its perfect and lonely hidden world is applicable to us as we are invited to open our hearts to start living in the present. It is an offer of grace to realize that life does not have to be perfect and that we should enjoy the world as it is being perfected. When we focus solely on building a perfect life, we fail in living today.

We have to open our ears so we can hear the sacred invitation to join in the game. We have to embrace the imperfections and finality of everything in life and appreciate the fact that we are part of a game which includes getting dirty. We miss the opportunity to experience the grace that nurtures and the beauty in creation when we fail to participate in this fun because we want to remain neat and clean. The trials we face daily are real, but instead of avoiding them, we must face them with grace if we hope to conquer them.

Inspired by New Beginnings

The suffering we face in life can be considered a test or trial. Sickness, pain, hunger, and death are trials. Those trials create a bridge for trust and expose our imperfections. The trials of life could help us see what we need to improve in our lives. Trials also help to show our strength and resiliency. It boosts our competency and reliance when we overcome obstacles. One of the greatest ways in which humanity has continued the indoctrination of the species is through education. While receiving our education, we have to prove that we understand and retain what we are taught. Unfortunately, the more we are able to memorize, the better students we are. To prove that we are educated, we have to be tested.

As kids, we grow up learning by trying things out on our own. We fail, we rebuild, and we try again. We succeed and fail again. We are never deterred from trying because of failure. We just fail and try again and again—and again and again. We are never limited by time as we have no concept of it. We try for hours to conquer the obstacles we face. These things may not be important to grown-ups, but for us, they are the only focal point. We sometimes laugh at our mistakes; at others, we cry but try again. We are never ashamed. When we achieve one milestone, we are inspired to conquer another. As we gain a level in the game, we try higher ones. This is how our lives evolve in the learning process until we are taught through a set of regulations, tests, and trials. Overcoming these set rules becomes our education.

Like with education, without these tests and trials, it would be difficult to show competency. The trials we face in life are like going through educational tests in preparation for a higher plane. We pass or we fail tests on a daily basis. We are tested by society, by family, friends, workplace, and the devil. We are tested by crisis, sickness, epidemics, and catastrophic experiences. While we are in this world, so many expectations are placed on us knowingly or unknowingly. We live trying to fulfil these expectations. At times, the trials of life do not allow us time to live. We solve one problem after another, and we fail to live in grace and fruitfulness. The tests and trials we go through in life prepare us for what we may face in the future. They could serve as distractions or tools to grow and as the foundation for us to be strong for future glory. "For now, we see only a reflection as in a mirror; then we shall see face to face. Now I know in part; then I shall know fully, even as I am fully known" (1 Corinthians 13:12).

Live Today, Hope for the Future

One day I went to see a patient. As I knocked and stepped into his room for a visit, the patient saw me and moaned. I was startled and didn't know what to say or do. I felt that he must have thought I was there for Last Rites because he noticed that I was wearing my priestly robe. I told him not to worry and that I was there to pray for his recovery and not to give him Last Rites. Despite my reassurance to him, he cried. That really touched me. I thought that something serious must have been causing a man in his late sixties or seventies to cry like that. I grabbed a chair and sat down by his bed and listened.

The patient narrated that he was intensely upset both with himself and God. He had received the most devastating news from the doctors. He had retired a month before and had a party with friends and family for his retirement. He had worked for his company for more than forty years. He was steadfast in his job and had made sacrifices that helped the company grow. The company hired him as a consultant for two additional years after retirement, and he went back to help. Finally, he retired, and his friends had a party to honor him. During this party, one of his friends suggested that he check with his doctor as his eyes looked yellow.

His wife had asked him several times in the past to go check with the doctor. He never felt it was necessary as his six months' checkup was coming up. He told his friend not to worry that he was feeling fine. One day he came back home, and his wife insisted he had to go to the hospital as he was not looking good. He wanted to brush it off and go the next day, but she insisted and started to cry. There was nothing else he could do but go to the doctor's. The doctor asked him to be admitted for them to run more tests. That was when he suspected something was wrong. The doctor had just given him the test results. He was told that his liver was failing. It was too late for him to have a liver transplant.

"I am not afraid of dying," he cried. "I know if I die, I will go to heaven. What hurts most is that I worked my entire life. Now that I could rest after retiring, be with my wife, family, and friends and enjoy the rewards of my labor, I hear that I am dying. Is this what God is paying me back with? It was painful for me to hear this news because I have not really 'lived' before going to heaven. I only worked and served others. My heart is broken because I feel cheated. I did not enjoy all the things I should have enjoyed in life. I worked, did things right, helped those in need, gave money to help the poor and I practiced my faith in God. I feel terrible because I failed to enjoy the good things. I was out there serving and building up this amazing financial company. It is now successful, but I lost *me* in the process. I lost time being with my family. I lost spending time with my wife. I lost going on vacation. I lost being one with nature and going swimming, hunting, and hiking.

"I invested it all—my life, money, and everything to build this company. Now I am at the hospital after all that work and the money I made. I feel ashamed because I saved every penny I made. I did not allow my wife to spend money on new clothes, except when she got them on sale. I avoided going to any restaurant to eat so as not to spend money unnecessarily. I never went to the concerts or movies that I wanted because I was not prepared to spend *that kind* of money. I used my old car for more than twenty years and managed every penny I made. It was only after my retirement that I decided for the first time in my life to buy a new truck. I prayed to God and asked, 'Please give me ten years! Please, even if it is only five, let me just have a life and spend it with my wife and family before I die.'

"I could feel my own pain, struggles, fears, worries, and brokenness as I listened to his. My mind was swirling with so many questions about my own regrets and failures. Did I fail to live my own life and lived only for others? Was I only working and failed and missed out on the most important thing of life—living? How many times in my ministry did I just do what I was told because of fear of not doing the right thing? How many times did I just obey the authorities and quieted the distinctiveness of my voice? Did I serve others while forgetting myself? Did I utilize all the graces God has given me? How often did I fail to appreciate and live in the moment? How many times did I get stuck in doing what is right instead of living my life? Did I worry too much about what people thought and said that I failed to be me? Did I miss the opportunity to laugh, dance, joke, and do what will give me joy because of what people might say? Did I receive blessings for myself or judge myself as self-centered? Did I block the voices of judgement accusing me of selfishness, insensitivity, and being uncaring when I did something I liked? Did I overburden myself with guilt? Did I fail to live today while I aspired for tomorrow? The list of these questions is endless."

A friend sent me this quote by Nanea Hoffman, "None of us are getting out of here alive, so please stop treating yourself like an afterthought. Eat the delicious food. Walk in the sunshine. Jump in the ocean. Say the truth you're carrying in your heart like hidden treasure. Be silly. Be kind. Be weird. There's no time for anything else."—Nanea Hoffman

This patient's life may be linked to the story of the man robbed and beaten up by thieves on his way to Jericho as Jesus narrated in the Bible. If he knew he was to be robbed, there was no way he would have embarked on that journey or followed that route. On this business trip, he was hoping to make more money. He took risks and hoped it would work out. Using the shorter route would have saved him in expenses. The thieves ambushed him and beat him up and took everything he had. Everything he had with him—all the money he borrowed, all the gold, and all the things he had worked—for were stripped from him on that journey. He was left on that route badly beaten and near death. Before this man was met by the Good Samaritan, everyone who passed by him left him to his fate.

Doctor reports at the hospital could be traumatic and life-changing for us. It may sound like being robbed and stripped of everything that makes us human. This man in tears and anguish in this hospital bed was clearly like the man on the road to Jericho—robbed, beaten, and abandoned by the robbers. This man felt that the doctor's report had stripped him of any happiness, joy, or hope for the future. He was already told he only had a few months to live. He laid in bed feeling abandoned, irredeemably broken, and left to die by God. He was in pain because of the guilt, his regrets, and anguish over never utilizing the time he had to live. He was hoping for a recompense and relaxation as a reward for retirement. Unfortunately, the expectation of this good life was short-lived. He lived all his life investing in the future while failing to live in the moment. He felt that his illness had robbed him of his humanity. He was angry and furious with himself, God, and everyone around. He was overwhelmed with regret, guilt, and felt ashamed that he had failed to live his life with his family while making money. He had focused on strategic planning for his future only. He failed to live and appreciate the gift of today. Missing those graces of today was a great source of grief and anguish in his heart.

Take a vacation and go on holidays when it can be afforded. Appreciate the beauty and blessings in the world within your means. It is okay to relax, celebrate life, and be thankful every day of our lives. However, we must reach out and help those in need. We have a responsibility to care for ourselves and others around us. Many people who are financially rich are broken and suffering just as everyone else. They may hide behind their money and flamboyancy. We are tempted to assume that all that glitters is indeed gold when the opposite is true. It is only when we get closer that we realize that they may not suffer financial hardship but that they also hurt and feel depleted. They share the same human ailments plaguing all of us—sickness, pain, fear, addiction, humiliation, and loneliness. Unfortunately, money and popularity can place us on pedestals and create the illusion that we are living above others. This creates distance between us and our loved ones and could cause separation from them. The result is emptiness and loneliness even in the age of 'in real time' communication. No amount of money or fancy gadgets can fill the gap created by the lack of personal connection.

Life is good, but it could be cruel, and we are limited in terms of what we can do about it. Many things are difficult to comprehend in the world we live in. It is in this category that I see pain as brokenness in times when we feel powerless. What could be done when we are faced with difficulties in our lives? What options do we have? It is in this mysterious moment that the melody "kpuu kpuu kpo ogene" comes handy. We have to walk back and experience the childhood that we lost and reclaim the authenticity of our being. We are invited to do this because life is precious and filled with grace. No one knows what will happen tomorrow. Reclaiming the simplicity of childlike trust would go a long way in offering us sustenance in times of difficulty. Once we reclaim this trust, we are able to discover the grace that God is revealing to us. "But when he, who from my mother's womb had set me apart and called me through his grace was pleased to reveal his Son to me" (Galatians 1:15).

During the time I was with this retiree, my heart went out to him for all those regrets and the pain he harbored in his heart. When people are suffering, what we say to them matters. There are times when it is better to keep quiet and not say anything. It is better than regurgitating things that every other person says. That may hurt the patient more than if we kept our mouths shut. If I told this man, "Whatever happens, happens for a reason," or "Have faith in God because you are a child of God, and God loves you!" or "At least now you know, and you can prepare yourself for heaven because heaven is the glorious place God prepared for those who love Him, you are going to heaven!"—how do you think he would feel? Would he feel supported? Would he feel strengthened in his struggle or discouraged and overwhelmed? How does heaven being "a better place" bring comfort to him? He does not want God to deliver him from this corrupt world yet. Does God really want him to come immediately to heaven because heaven is better than earth? Saint Paul says, "Eyes have not seen, ears have not heard, now does it enter the mind of humanity what God has prepared to those who love him" (1 Corinthians 2:9).

God is the one who supports us in our own faith journey so we can journey with others in their suffering.

> Praise be to God, the Father of our Lord Jesus Christ, the Father of mercies, and the God of all consolation! He comforts us in all our afflictions enabling us to comfort those who are in trouble, with the same consolation we have received from him. As we have shared much in the suffering of Christ, so through Christ do we share abundantly in his consolation. (2 Corinthians 1:3–5)

God is the one who will make our burden light if we take it to Him in prayer.

The Past Is Irreversible, Living Is Not

I felt that the patient's cry was not only the pain of becoming sick. His regret stemmed from the fact that he had failed to *live*. He was bemoaning the loss of the life that he had failed to live. He had made money and worked for others and could not be there for himself. Pope John Paul II said, "Through work man must earn his daily bread and contribute to the continual advance of science and technology." Earning our daily bread should never be at the expense of our lives, and neither should they infringe upon our freedom. We have to make every effort so that we are not chained by work or money.

This man's condition and situation were heartbreaking. His experience could happen to anyone of us any day and anytime. Our plans could change instantly because of sickness. We are never in control of our lives or health. We are never sure of what the future has in store for us. We could do everything humanly possible to protect and provide for ourselves, but we are not really 100 percent in control of our health. God has the final say. He is the Creator of the universe who is always there for us to see Him all around us. Without the grace of God, there was nothing meaningful or reasonable I could offer him. I just sat there and prayed in my heart while I allowed him to continue to cry. I stayed with him in silence as he expressed his fears. I continued to pray silently in my heart, and after a long while and with a heavy heart I said to him, "There are no words in this world that can provide comfort to you at this time after the type of news you received. You have to give yourself the grace to understand why you feel the way you do right now. I am not here to take away the pain and tell you that everything is going to be okay. I am here to share this time of difficulty with you. I am here to pray with you and ask for God's intervention in this suffering. Above all, I pray that God would give you the grace to bear this pain well." Honestly, I was not sure why God had placed me there with him.

I told him, "There is nothing anyone can do about the past. The future—that is all we have today. We could retell our own stories instead of allowing others to do that for us. The future is right now." I asked him, "If you have days, weeks, months or years to live, what would you do? I can't imagine how stressful this is for you right now. Nothing I can say will bring back lost times. You can either make every second you have left in life count or use every second to focus on the regrets of the past in terms of failed expectations."

I wish to reiterate that missed opportunities to live happen when we focus on building a better future and fail to live today. We have to build the future, but it should not be to the detriment of living fully today. Yesterday and tomorrow are all part of our lives. What is important is the value of what we have today. We will become selfish and self-centered if *we* and what we want is all that matters. That is narcissistic and destructive to human existence because no one is an island. We have to live today and join others who are on this journey with us. Our daily living and the little things we do are what become extraordinary. It is useless to save all the money for the future if we fail to live in the moment as we build for the future. We should learn that tomorrow is inseparable from today. We live today as we build for the future. We cannot live fixated on the mistakes of the past. We cannot live terrified and hiding from the shadows of the past. We have to learn! We adjust as we hope for greater heights.

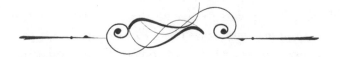

Transforming Helplessness

A hospitalization limits our capacity to do so many things we loved to do. Everyone dreads the loss of independence. Yet the first thing we freely sign off on when we enter the hospital for treatment is our freedom. We give up our freedom to do whatever we want, move around as we want, eat what we want, and determine who enters our room. Once we set foot in the hospital environment for treatment, we lose our independence. This experience of dependence on others when sick means others control us and tell us what to do. Whether we like it or not, the sicker we are, the more our bodies become frail, the more we are dependent on others, and this makes our spirits feeble. This challenge of dependence on others because of our limitations could make us feel incapacitated, worthless, and of no use. The experience of stagnancy could be stressful, disorienting, and frustrating because it makes us feel we are a burden. Irrespective of whatever may be happening when we are sick, we get to control one gift only, and that is our attitude. How we choose to respond and deal with the enormous challenge of losing control of our authority is a manifestation of grace. The attitude we consciously convey to others in sickness is our personal choice, irrespective of the pain we go through. That is the power that we have to either use it well or not. We may not have all the abilities we used to before becoming sick, but how do we use the tiniest power we still have?

While in the hospital, we receive care and love from strangers as we hope to recover. We are practically dependent on the nurses for our hygiene, using the bathroom, getting up from bed, and lying down. We always feel we should be helping others. Depending on others is a mark of laziness and weakness. We believe we have a duty to take care of others, and we struggle when the reality becomes that we are to receive care. We do feel horribly because of this inability to help and do things for others. In this state of discomfort and dependence, are we aware that we have some great gifts that we could use even in our diminished condition? Do we know that although we may be very sick, we do not have a monopoly on suffering? Our attitude definitely will change toward others as they provide us with care. Are we sensitive to the fact that those caring for us are also human? Do we know we all have something we are dealing with even when we do not advertise it for all to see? Could we dig deeper into the depths of our being to find out those things still in us that we may share with others to make a difference? Every human being we meet struggles with something, professionally or otherwise, and may not show it. Do we realize we are writing our story of love and kindness in the hearts of all those nurses, doctors, and all who walk into our hospital room trying to care for us? We are either blessing them or piercing their hearts and wounding them more.

Jesus, in the Gospel of Luke, told the story of observing those putting their gifts into the temple treasury. Above all those who donated generously, a poor widow with two pennies was Jesus's pick. Jesus said the woman gave more than every other person because she gave everything she had (Luke 21:1–4). This woman deliberately walked in with only two pennies. She gave all she had and went home with nothing. While not using this story as a sermon, it brings to mind the grace of the gifts we have. This story of the widow could serve as an example to redefine what scarcity means for us at the hospital.

Like this widow, we should accept our limitations but treasure our blessings while we are at the hospital. Limitations are not things to be ashamed of. They energize us to make optimal and generous use of scarce resources. When it comes to utilizing grace, numbers do not matter. It is our ability to look beyond quantity and lay claim to the incredible entrails of grace in scarcity. It is only with this blessing that we allow limitation to stand up for itself and not be muddled up in shame for not being enough. How are we able to sow seeds with what we have instead of waiting till we get everything we think we deserve, want, or need. Would that be enough? Converting limitations to useful output is how we can manifest God's grace. This story of the widow's mite can mirror the hospital experience. While in the hospital, we are limited in our capabilities and resources. Do we remember that everyone we meet is broken and hurting in one way or another? Are we their angel of light, or do we present ourselves as their crosses? Could we find out our own two pennies and use them to minister to those who are broken and hurting like we are?

One Saturday, I went for my routine rounds to visit Catholic patients at the hospital for anointing of the sick. I went to the hospital hurting because I had received a message stating that a patient I met had died. I had prayed and hoped she was recovering and doing better, but it obviously did not happen as I had hoped. She was being buried that day. I was not able to attend her funeral that morning because I had a presentation to give, and I couldn't find anyone to replace me. At about 4:00 p.m., almost at the end of my visits, I was really tired. I had one more patient to visit, and my mind was still filled with sorrow due to the news of her death. I was dragging my feet to the last visit. (I know that as a priest, everyone expects us to be strong, stoic, and not show any sign of tiredness because, after all, we are God's messengers. I laugh because people do not connect human emotions to the expected life of "church" and "priestly" life). I entered a room and saw that the patient, a young woman, was in agonizing pain. I wanted to leave immediately and come back another day. Even in her agonizing pain, she was very pleasant and welcomed me with a smile and said, "Father, sorry I am in terrible pain right now. It is not a good time to see me. Thank you for coming, and please pray for me before you leave."

That splendid smile and warmth she showed me was something extraordinary. I could not take it for granted. I was in awe looking at her in such a horrible pain and still reaching out to welcome me with this smile. I said brief prayers for her, and I allowed her to rest. I thanked her for blessing me because I felt blessed and touched by her inner strength to welcome me as she had, even in the horrible pain she was in. As I was greeting her mother and about to leave, she screeched in pain. I could not pretend that I hadn't heard it. I could not leave while she was in such a state. I watched as the mother and their friend supported and comforted her. As I waited and she became calm, she still thanked me again with the depth of sincere beauty and appreciation, which made me feel energized as I left to go home. I told her that she had made my day even in the midst of her pain. I really appreciated her blessing me with her gift of love and smile. I went home refreshed and replenished with her simple gesture of allowing the abundance of grace to flow in such brokenness.

This young woman was stressed because of a rare disease that caused her great pain in her spinal cord. Yet in such pain, she went out of her way to welcome me because I had gone to pray for her. She transformed her pain into a blessing and moment of grace to bless me. Like the widow's mite, she still found her two coins even while in pain and lacking anything else to offer. She blessed me and so many other staff members who walked into her room, tired, weak, and weary with her bright smile. She converted her lack into resources and changed the narrative of scarcity and pain to plenitude. No matter how little our coin may appear to us, it is still gold. The value is found in the quality and not quantity. Sharing that limitedness is the gift and blessings of abundance. What is our own widow's mite that will be of benefit to those feet who walk into our hospital rooms or who cross our daily paths?

What do we have that we could willingly give up and put into the treasury? Like the story of the allegory I shared, the young men in the cave only saw pebbles. They never opened their bags till they got home to see that they had gold all along. We have to start looking deeper to see that hidden in the depth of our being is beautiful, precious gold. We should see that hidden in us is beauty and grace and not weakness, sickness, and old burdens. In times of need, grace helps us to be creative to use the pebble as is to turn it into gold. Grace helps us to create other possibilities even beyond our imagination instead of settling for less. We should recognize that the pebbles are not just pebbles but gold and that we are not to leave them in the cave. The story of the widow's mite is finding abundance in scarcity and limitations. It is turning our little resources into an abundance of blessings to be shared with others. It is rewriting our story of suffering and transforming it to make a difference.

Amplifying Our Dignity

St. Thomas Aquinas said in Latin, "*Gratia non tollit naturam, sed perficit.*" "Grace does not destroy nature, grace perfects nature," or "Grace does not remove nature but fulfills it." Grace does not function in a void or emptiness. It is built on what is available. There is a gift given to each and every one of us from birth. We may feel that the gifts are not enough, and we want more. We have to be careful so that we understand that what is important is planting the seeds that we are given and using them. The seeds cannot multiply if we do not help them grow. Jesus, in the story of the talents, tells us of three servants given different talents. One of them, because he felt the talent he received was too little compared with others, buried it instead of trading with it (Matthew 25:14–30). Unlike the servant who buried his talents because he felt he did not have enough, the story of the poor widow displays the power of utilizing scarcity and turning it into abundance.

In our hospital experiences, it feels like we are being emptied of everything we have—our capacities, our tastes, our freedom, and everything we used to rely on. While at the hospital, we wear nothing except for the shapeless hospital gown that everyone wears, both male and female. Actually, nothing stopped this poor widow from focusing on her gift instead of on her lack. She must have felt self-conscious wearing her modest dress walking through the isle of the temple, but that did not stop her. She knew how special the occasion was, and her lack did not prevent her from moving forward to offer what gifts she had: her two coins. How do we face the situations we encounter with courage and grace? How do we accept the reality of the pain we are going through and not shame the experience or become wrapped up in the "pity me" and "poor me" mentality? "Those who know your name trust in you, for you, Lord have never forsaken those who seek you" (Psalm 9:10).

The poor widow, in her scarcity, offered the last thing she had, thus depending entirely on God by giving the gift of her two small coins. While others were living and giving in abundance, she lived in lack and gave the entirety of her scarce resources. Jesus saw the enormity of her small gift and praised her. Remember that coins make noise when dropped on the metal dish. In this temple, some of her husband's friends would have very likely been present to give their showy donations. Yet she was courageous to drop her two coins, aware that they would make little to no noise. It would have been easier for her to save herself the embarrassment of seeing her husband's friends watch her in humiliation while they enjoyed their wealth. Thank goodness she didn't focus on the pain, resentment, and bitterness that she must have felt after everything had been taken away from her. If she had focused on that, she would not have gone to the temple or walked through the isle. She offered what little she had in abundance and grace.

At the hospital, it is easy to focus on our lack and limitations by accepting the inevitable: powerlessness. We lose our freedom, our choices of food, and our ability to move around and help others. Therefore, we have nothing to offer because we are in pain and suffering, or so we think. That is not really the case. It is really not true that we have nothing. We have something, no matter how small we think it may be. We may have lived believing the lies that we were made to believe over the years: that we have nothing to offer. Those lies disempower us because we feel terrible and not well enough, thus giving up in making even the smallest of efforts. A woman once told me how she stood up for herself: "I have been a nurse for more than forty years. I am sick, and I know that, but I cannot trade my respect and dignity for anything. I stood up for myself and insisted that they bring me food since they cancelled my surgery. I didn't hear from them for more than two hours. I asked my nurse, and she said they were still on it. I kept on looking at the time. After an hour, I called her again and told her how I felt about her negligence and nonchalant attitude. She apologized, and within a few minutes, I got the food. It felt good to realize that even though I was sick, I did not accept that type of neglect."

Remember that grace opens our eyes to see our inner being and appreciate our two coins as gold and learn to offer them to God as blessings. The experience of searching deeper and presenting what we have is the grace of abundance. We have to offer what we have, be it the jar of oil and flour as the widow of Zarephath, finding our two coins like the story of the widow, or bringing more pebbles as in the young men with gold who thought they had pebbles. We should value our voice, our identity, and our being for who we are. We ought to appreciate our distinctiveness as a blessing and not in competition with others. Humility does not involve humiliation or having to feel inferior to others. We are God's children and creation. We are beautifully created and made to be distinct in His grace. He wants our total dependence on His providence and conviction that He will take care of us. Living in scarcity and living in grace are two different things. This poor widow Jesus used as an example is saying that she had nothing left to live on. Whatever it was, she only had one life to live. She chose to live in the abundance of the day and give all she had to it. This offering of herself completely without reservation is what opens us up to receive the abundance of grace.

Defying the Logic of Scarcity

We have an innate desire to help and support others when they are in need. When we are admitted to the hospital, we are not able to do much to help others. The hospital makes us face our limitations. The experience may make us feel lonely, abandoned, neglected, devoid of energy, and helpless. We tend to focus on our limitations and scarcity. What if we focused on those gifts that even sickness cannot take away from us? Grace manifests itself when we reclaim the good in our life. It happens when we refuse to hand over the remote control of our attitude to sadness and hopelessness while leaning on our Lord for support. "I will praise you, for I am fearfully and wonderfully made" (Psalm 139:14).

Defying the reality of limitation was exemplified by David in his fight against Goliath. David was a young lad. He was inexperienced in the act of war and fighting. He was by no means equal to Goliath, a trained warrior who had been in numerous battlefields and defeated his enemies. When it mattered most, David did not depend on the shield and the tools provided to him by the soldiers. He relied on his own insight and grace. He faced Goliath as he was with his limited resources and won the fight (1 Samuel 17). Overcoming Goliath is clearly the plight of so many patients at the hospital.

I once met a woman suffering from diabetes who was to undergo a double leg amputation. I was astonished to witness the amazing comforting spirit she had. In the course of our conversations, she shared all her fears about her surgery in a fun sort of way that had us in stitches. She explained that it was devastating to hear that she needed the amputation but that she had accepted it after a while. She did not allow others to narrate her story for her. She chose to own her story and told them how she felt. She spiced her fears with a healthy dose of fun and joked that she was joining the "privileged class." I didn't understand what she meant until she explained that while everyone else fights for a parking spot at the grocery store, Black Friday sales, or Christmas shopping, she was going to be able to pull right into the handicapped parking. "Thank God it is not my fingernails they are getting rid of. At least I will still be able to fix my nails." I thought to myself, *Are you serious? With everything that you have on your plate, you are thinking about your nails?* It felt strange that her nails were that important to her. She smiled and said, "Now I will be able to sit down and relax as I ask my husband, 'Bring the milk! Get the cheese, and—I don't like that one, get yogurt, and now that you are on it, bring the strawberries too!'" The husband was sitting there and just laughed.

She turned her fears and worry into jokes and fun to cope with the enormity of it all. She joked about the shock her old friends would get after seeing her without legs. She mimicked how she would laugh watching the look of shock in their faces. She imagined how her pants would dangle beneath her knees after the amputation. She had definitely been blessed with this incredible sense of humor.

I visited her again a few times to pray with her and offer support. In one of those visits, we had a deeper conversation, and I was surprised when she told me about her main fear about her new condition. She was shocked at the news, and she feared she would become a burden to her family. She was afraid the amputation would change her life and that she was going to be permanently dependent on others. She found grace for herself through the light of God's

Holy Spirit while she prayed and cried. As she came to accept what her future was going to be, she turned her fears and worries of being a burden to the family into jokes. She accepted the reality of the new lifestyle as well as its inevitability.

> God has a sense of humor, and I am finding my own. It was devastating to hear that my feet would be gone while I lived. It was depressing. The news of the amputation was the saddest news of my life. Losing my feet was like losing my beauty. To me, it was losing who I was and my identity. Why do my feet have to be removed so I can live? I do not really understand. After the news, I was so devastated and angry that I went to God for answers. I went to church and prayed. As I prayed, I asked God for healing and a miracle. I honestly felt broken, and in my brokenness, I felt His presence. I heard this silent voice, *I am with you. I will take you where you could never imagine. Your suffering has no final say, for I am the Alpha and the Omega, the beginning and the end.* That day, I saw God's light shine in my heart as it enveloped me. I cried for hours as I prayed. After this experience, I had this inexplicable peace in my heart, and my spirit exploded with joy. Amputating my feet would not amputate my joy or who I am. I not only came to accept that, but I was joyous, trusting God. I had felt that life was over for me. I heard a voice say to me, *I am with you, and you have so many things to offer to the world.* Since then, I have felt different. I have become more open to the new graces God is giving me. I do not feel terrible about being a burden to my family. I served others in the past and would willingly do that again if I could. I am not going to deny others the opportunity to be

God's channel of love and service. That is how
I see my life. I am learning to trust God, and I
accept the love and support I receive from my
family and friends.

She hopes to continue teaching dance classes as she waits to see
what God has in store for her. She smiled as she talked and had a look
of inner joy. She chose not to give up because she would have no feet.
She planned to have a new life, train herself to read music, sing and
play the piano in her church. She felt that losing her feet was opening
many new possibilities for her to explore. The amputation was not
going to determine the outcome of her life. She would fight and find
life for herself despite losing what she uses most in her everyday life.
She succeeded in turning her loss into gold. She was able to find her
two coins for herself and offered them without being ashamed of her
limitations. Her broad smile and laughter were always contagious,
and she did not want anyone to pity her. Healing for her did not
mean avoiding the amputation but that she had found a new light
for herself. God healed her without changing her circumstances. He
healed her by being with her as she turned her cross into glory and
wealth. She reclaimed the abundance of her graces.

The Distinctiveness of Our Gift

In valuing the gift God gives us, one thing we must always
remember is that our two coins belong to us. We are not perfect,
and God is only perfecting us. We primarily trust His mercy, love,
and grace. Saint Paul states, "You are God's masterpiece" (Ephesians
2:10). Each and every one of us, though distinct, is a masterpiece
designed by the Divine Master. So we should always remember that
our coins are never the same as another person's. We make the mistake of comparing our graces with those of others. What is my own
gift and grace? Am I comfortable with that, or am I waiting and
expecting something different? This gift of distinctiveness is what
grace is helping us to realize. When we live in grace, we are no longer held back by people's expectations of us. We find our own voice

while appreciating the respective gifts every other person has to offer. Many times, we are so distracted playing roles and doing what people expect of us that we lose the sacredness of our distinctiveness. It is always important to remember that we are who we are. We should not worry about being like another person. There is always something more in us when we tap into the depth of our being. "May your unfailing love be my comfort, according to your promise to your servant" (Psalm 119:76).

To look after those who are sick, weak, old, and challenged and find peace is possible only through the grace and mercy of God. Everyone in this ministry is broken and shares in the brokenness. The distinctiveness of our gift is that both patient and caregivers have something to offer in bringing healing to the sacred space for healing. We all need the healing touch of God, whether we are the patient or caregiver. Hospitals become a place where we are all invited to a fellowship of healing. It is never too small a gesture to stretch our hand out and bless those who enter our room with a faint smile even when in pain. Caregivers can help us find deeper meaning in our work and ministry. It is only in the eyes of grace that we can find God in those we care for day and night. Through grace, wiping a patient or loved ones' lips would be like Veronica wiping Jesus's face as He experienced excruciating pain. Appreciating our distinctiveness will help us serve one another with love and grace. We would understand that we are Jesus's hands and feet, anointing one another with healing oil and love.

There is deeper beauty in the journey of finding out that our coins are gold. We have to creatively determine how to best use the precious gifts we have so that with the true light of grace, we can see their true value. It matters not the size of our gift but how we invest what we have and make perfect use of it. We are more than enough for the master who made us exactly as we are. We have to be like the widow who had the audacity to come out with all she had and unlike the young men blinded by greed. We should not hesitate to use our God-given gift, even if it is only the gift of a smile.

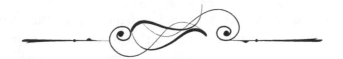

Modifying Our Worldviews

In our world, the probability of our encountering suffering is 100 percent. It is also comforting that God gives us 100 percent of His grace to face it. Witnessing suffering is unavoidable. We encounter it either directly or indirectly, but it is an unavoidable part of our existence. We see our friends or family members suffering or hear about children dying, wars, hunger, fire, and flooding. Our hearts go out to those who suffer, and we do share in their pain. The road we travel is paved with pitfalls, wants, lacks, distractions, temptations, sickness, and so much more. Everything we do in this world could be in preparation for that ultimate destiny for which we were made. The ultimate goal is to unite our suffering with God's will in perfect unity to behold His glory. There is no shortcut in life to achieve our purpose of connecting to glory without sacrifice and suffering. As we face the reality of suffering, God made us strong and poured His graces on us so we could withstand temptation. We are on a journey to our ultimate destination, which is the highest glory that is to be revealed after our journey on earth.

Everyone we meet, irrespective of what image they portray, struggles. They may not always come to us to announce it, but we all have our share of suffering. We have crosses to bear, be it sickness, disease, drug addiction, alcohol, no job, poverty—the list is endless. Everywhere we go, every office we enter, and every job we do, we can see people struggling in different ways. "Be alert and of sober mind. Your enemy the devil prowls around like a roaring lion looking for someone to devour" (1 Peter 5:8). What is our response in times of temptation and persecution? Do we fight to defend ourselves? Are we not required to turn the other cheek as Jesus Christ taught us? How do we reconcile accepting our sickness as the will of God and praying for God's healing power? Many saints handed over their suffering to God in atonement for the suffering of others and the sins of the world. Are we not supposed to see our suffering as the will of God and accept it as the saints did?

During my year of residency for the Clinical Pastoral Education program in 2018, I was once called to be present while a family was trying to make an end of life decision. The doctors told the family that the patient was in an irreversible condition and would never recover. The family was informed that they had the choice as to when they wanted the machines to be turned off as the patient was actively dying. I sat there, hearing all these things, and asked myself, what would I do if I had to make such a decision? I felt the pain and fear in the hearts of everyone in this family. As the meeting progressed, I asked the doctor for permission to allow the family time to process the information and make their decision. This moment and space allowed them to stop the clock for a moment and simply breathe. As I walked out, the father followed me and thanked me for the brief moment they had. He said he was afraid to make the decision about someone else's life. "I do not feel I can do this. I know he is my son, but I am not God, and He is the only one who can decide who lives or dies. I am conflicted about turning life support off for my child."

This man's struggle was an eye-opener. I witnessed the painful reality of the young man actively dying. The family was terrified of "giving up" on their son and on any further efforts that could potentially save his life. They had faith and hoped for a miracle, but it did look as if nothing else could be done. I told the man that this was a really difficult time. I pointed out to him that once everything that could possibly have been done is done, it is okay to grant dignity to the dying person. For me, it was no longer an issue of right or wrong, but in that painful moment, it was allowing a loved one to go with honor and peacefully. We have to be strong to express our love for the person. Being strong does not mean not crying. Tears are not a sign of weakness as we may be led to believe. Tears are a way of expressing our deep-felt love. The guilt of turning off the machine was only one aspect of the decision. The knowledge that with a flick of a switch there would be no life left in him was even worse. However, we may hesitate to make the decision and unknowingly prolong the pain just because it is harder to let go. Allowing nature to take its course when we have done everything possible may be a merciful way of bidding farewell to the person we love. A few weeks later, someone in the store walked up to me. He reminded me that I had recently been with him at the hospital when his son was dying. He thanked me for what I had done for them that day and told me that I had helped them deal with their pain and fears.

As humans, we are endowed with the capacity to make decisions and choices based on our free will. When we fail to make the best decisions, the consequences are guilt and regret. While grief and regret may not necessarily be the solution, we should not minimize the importance of regretting mistakes. We are not supposed to dwell on our mistakes and hold ourselves chained to guilt. We ought to move on and learn from them and consider them as opportunities to grow and receive grace. We do have a responsibility to hold ourselves accountable and avoid getting distracted from God's plan for us. Acknowledging and accepting our mistakes are the very essence of grace. What opportunity for grace did I miss? What graces did I waste that I need to reclaim? The future rests on the foundations laid yesterday and the ones we are laying now. The future, yesterday, and today are all held together by grace and are inseparable. We have the opportunity to move from past mistakes by God's grace, by the grace of others, and by giving ourselves grace. There is always a second chance.

For generations, humanity has attempted to find answers to understand the origin of human suffering. Many cultures developed different reasons to explain failure, war, famine, epidemics, and diseases. Suffering must have an origin and must be caused by something. One of the easiest approaches, in absence of an obvious answer, was the belief that humanity was affected by God. God was to them a completely independent and all-powerful, mysterious being. He did not stop calamities affecting human beings rendering them powerless in the face of evil. In an effort to solve crises, humans decided that the best course of action was to appease these all-powerful gods.

Whatever request was made by the gods were immediately fulfilled in order to end pandemonium. Even when the demands were absurd, people still had to carry them out to save the whole community. This meant sacrificing animals, money, humans, and even children. In some cultures, to give birth to twins was considered a taboo, and the newly born kids were sacrificed to appease the gods and save the community from the wrath of these deities. This ruthlessness was justified and seen as the will of the gods.

As we look around, we ask, What did we do wrong? Is there a connection between sin and suffering or diseases? Why does God allow children to suffer from a genetic disease that was never their fault? Did we do anything in the past for which God is punishing us? What unforgivable sin did we commit? He forgave others; why is our sin unforgiveable? We are ready to ask for forgiveness from Him. "God our Savior, for the glory of your name; deliver us and forgive our sins for your name's sake. Why should the nations say, 'Where is their God?'" (Psalm 79:9–10).

We tremble in fear searching for meaning and answers in the face of suffering. There are times when we just surrender to our suffering. We feel it is our fate, and we try to justify it. This view is a way to anchor our fears. We search in the shadows of our past. We judge ourselves and determine that surely "this must be my fault." We are the ones who transgressed, and therefore, our suffering is justifiable. Because it is justifiable, we convince ourselves that we have to endure it in attrition for our sins. In the Old Testament, Judaism like every other religion in the Ancient Near East, attributed all suffering to punishments delivered from a higher being—God.

This view was aggressively passed on from generation to generation by well-meaning people. They extracted these teaching from different passages of the scriptures that could be interpreted to read as such. "Yet, he does not leave the guilty unpunished; he punishes the children and their children for the sin of the parents to the third and fourth generation" (Exodus 34:7). We also ask, is it the sins of our ancestors that He is punishing us for?

For no one is cast off by the Lord forever. Though he brings grief, he will show compassion, so great is his unfailing love. For he does not willingly bring affliction or grief to anyone…Who can speak and have it happen if the Lord has not decreed it? Is it not from the mouth of the Most High that both calamities and good things come? Why should the living complain when punished for their sins? Let us examine our ways and test them, and let us return to the Lord. Let us lift up our hearts and our hands to God in heaven, and say: "We have sinned and rebelled and you have not forgiven. You have covered yourself with anger and pursued us; you have slain without pity. You have covered yourself with a cloud so that no prayer can get through. You have made us scum and refuse among the nations." (Lamentations 3:31–45)

Actually, we desperately desire to have the answers that could address the source of our suffering. Having this understanding is a great source of comfort and consolation. We could find a scapegoat on whom to unleash our guilt to rid ourselves of blame. We try to find answers as to the source of our suffering. This aims to provide some sort of comfort and ultimately meaning to our suffering.

I visited a patient to pray for his recovery, and all he kept saying was what a terrible person he was. He emphasized that God was punishing him with disease for all the bad stuff he had done. "It is all my fault. God is paying me back for my past life. I committed terrible sins many years ago. That must be the reason why He has abandoned me."

It has also been claimed that our prayers are not answered because of our sins or the sins of our parents, as well as all ancestral sins. Truly, sin hinders, separates, and breaks our relationship with God, with our fellow humans, and other creation. However, when it comes to linking sin to suffering, Jesus distances Himself from that concept. When He addressed those who asked Him about the blind man, "Rabbi, who sinned, this man or his parents, that he was born blind?" Jesus replied, "Neither this man nor his parents sinned, but this happened so that the works of God might be displayed in him" (John 9:1–12). We also recall Jesus's answer when He was told about the Galileans whose blood Pilate had mixed with their sacrifices. He answered them, "Do you think that these Galileans were worse sinners than all the other Galileans because they suffered this way? I tell you, no! But unless you repent, you too will all perish. Or those eighteen who died when the tower in Siloam fell on them—do you think they were more guilty than all the others living in Jerusalem? I tell you, no!" God allows the rain to fall on the good and the bad. The just and the unjust (Matthew 5:48). He does not set apart His blessings only for those who are good. He gives everyone the opportunity to experience Him like He allows the sun to shine on us all.

The Shadow of Self-Judgement

It is important to know that no matter how many crises we face, they too will come to pass. Having a stroke, no matter how small, could be scary. The brain is the connecting center for every part of our body. If the brain ceases to function or work at full capacity, the result is paralysis of different parts of our body. If anything happens to the brain, it affects every part of our body more so than any other organ. Yet the brain cannot function without other parts of the body. Those other parts are no less important. Every part should be cared for as long as it is not to the detriment of the other parts.

Taking care of oneself is never an act of selfishness. Sometimes we feel selfish or self-centered when we take time for ourselves. We interpret Jesus's command to love our neighbor as ourselves as self-sacrifice. We make it appear that doing good for others is more valuable than being good to ourselves—as if our own lives were not as important as those of others. When we take proper care of ourselves, we appreciate the gift of God in us. It is then that we truly see and love our neighbor as ourselves. When we do not fully cherish our body as the temple of the Holy Spirit, care for it as God's holy temple, it is difficult to care for others and show our love for them.

Many of us struggle with "Catholic guilt" when we take a little time to care for ourselves or treat ourselves. (Catholic guilt is the judgement we exercise on ourselves by deeming everything around us that is pleasurable as sin. It is also when we see everything as falling into the category of sin either of omission or commission, and it blinds us to grace.) In this sense, we feel that anything enjoyable that we may do for ourselves is a sign of selfishness, greediness, and pride. This distracts us from heavenly goals. Even when, in theory, we do know that these things are not sinful, in practice, we feel the weight of guilt for not caring for others. So many times, we turn a blind eye to our own needs and focus on the needs of our children, parents, friends, and anyone else who may need us. When we do not fully care for ourselves, we are not really capable of reaching out and helping someone else. One of Saint Irenaeus of Lyons popular quotes states, "The glory of God is man fully alive." As humans, if we are fully alive, mentally, spiritually, and psychologically, we can make full use of our potential. The glory of God shines in every living human. That includes us too as God's living creatures. We cannot take care of the needs of others and forget ourselves in the process.

Remember, humility does not imply not caring for ourselves. It does not mean feeling that our needs are secondary and inferior to the needs of others. Saint Paul's teaching on humility is misinterpreted to imply that humility means that we think of others more than ourselves. Saint Paul says, "Do nothing out of selfish ambition or vain conceit. Rather, in humility value others above yourselves, not looking to your own interests but each of you to the interests of the others" (Philippians 2:3–4). C. S. Lewis said it best: "True humility is not thinking less of yourself; it is thinking of yourself less." What we are, in fact, encouraged to avoid is self-love, which leads to greed, self-centeredness, and selfishness.

While we feel we have a responsibility to care for others, we should never compromise our own needs and desires. If we are all created in the image and likeness of God, then each one of us is equally important before God. Being humble does not imply that our own life has less value than another person's life. As we try to help and solve the problems of every other person, we have the responsibility of extending grace to ourselves. Our well-being matters too. To understand that our own personal needs should never be taken for granted or belittled cannot be overemphasized. We should never treat ourselves as second-class citizens, and neither are we less important than others. That attitude is not a sign of humility. When we travel by plane, we are always reminded that in case of an emergency, the oxygen mask will drop and that we must place the mask over our faces before attempting to help a child or someone else. We cannot think or solve our problems when we are operating at 40 percent, let alone be of assistance to other people. Accusing or judging ourselves as selfish for looking after ourselves can be considered part of the lies that bombard us.

As much as we share this responsibility to care for ourselves, we should not look away to avoid the need of others. It is definitely selfishness when we do not share the resources we have to help out another person when they need our help and support. The popular quote in the Bible against the rich states, "But woe to you who are rich, for you have already received your comfort" (Luke 6:24). This means that Jesus is clearly condemning the arrogance of the rich when they take for granted their privilege and avoid responsibility. We all have to care for the needs of others. It is not about being materially rich but being wealthy. Wealth has to do with fullness of grace. It's the type of wealth that makes us feel satisfied and content with God's blessings. It is the arrogance in feeling above others due to our circumstances that needs to be avoided.

In Cana, Galilee, Jesus performed His first miracle by turning six jars of water into wine (John 2:1–12). He didn't turn it into soda but into good wine. Good wine is a source of joy, especially when not abused. This miracle is a testament to the fact that when we are in crisis, our Lord and Savior, Jesus Christ, is never happy to allow us to be humiliated by our circumstances. Jesus wants us to be happy. I hear Him say that He will deliver us in His own time. In this first miracle of Jesus, the bridegroom must have been scared and terrified when the news of the wine running out was brought to his attention.

I guess looking at the number of guests still waiting in line for wine, he must have felt utterly hopeless. He would have given up the hope of being able to do anything to salvage the situation. The bride might have even started to cry because of the shame. She would have been terrified to be mocked because her newly wedded husband was not capable of providing enough wine for her wedding. At a time when all hope had faded, Jesus came to their rescue. He asked the servants to fill six more jars with water. That is how God is. The groom must have sung like the psalmist, "You have changed my mourning into dancing, O Lord, and have girded me with joy. Alleluia!" (Psalm 30:12). I believe that one day our tears will be turned into laugher!

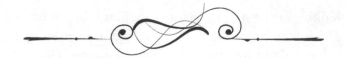

Humanity in Need of Grace

One day during my chaplaincy training program, I walked into a patient's room. I saw two guards sitting with a young man in the room. I observed the shackles on his feet. He was a prisoner. I was afraid and wanted to get out of the room as soon as I could. However, the patient wanted to talk. I sat and just listened to his life story. He said he had grown up in a terrible, poor neighborhood, and everyone he knew around the area was either in or had just come out of jail. Most of those who were released could not maintain a steady job or get any decent job because nobody wanted someone with a criminal record. In their neighborhood, those who were not in jail were in training to end up incarcerated, and it was only a matter of time till they graduated.

> My mom gave birth to me when she was fifteen, and she could not take care of me. She refused to give me up for adoption. She said it would break her heart if another person had to look after her child. One day, she was angry with me and told me that when I was born, there was no joy in her heart. Her eyes pierced me like I was her nemesis. She said she could not finish high school because of me and that my dad was sixteen at the time. He stole money from a gas station so he could pay for me to be aborted. The day they were scheduled to see the doctor for the abortion, the doctor was sick with the flu, and it took several weeks for him to get better. She made it sound like I had made the doctor sick. When the doctor

went back to work, my mother was scared to go back for the abortion. She was afraid she could die in the process. For several days, she fought with my biological dad, who insisted he would have nothing to do with the baby (me). After that, she informed her mom of her condition and about the decision she had made. She gave birth to me after the nine months. I have never heard my father's voice. My mom said he moved on with his life and told me his name. When I checked him out, he was serving a thirty-two-year prison sentence for murder.

Growing up, I had this dream of making a difference in the world. I hoped to make good money and buy a very good house for my momma. I was never going to allow her to suffer again after all she had been through in life. I wish I had a dad! I wish I had met my dad! I wish my dad was there to correct me and teach me what was right or wrong. I wish I had a dad of whom I could be afraid when I did something wrong and who would have punished me. I wish I had a dad that I could share my secrets with during puberty. I wish I had a dad who would have beaten me and shouted at me!

My head was spinning just listening to him.

Now the guards yell at me. I wish I had a dad who could create boundaries for me and given me time-outs. I am chained by police and guards. I have been to different prisons and cells. It would have been a great experience for me to hear the voice of my dad say, "Shut up! Don't say that."

My first jail sentence was when I was fourteen. I was angry with my mom's boyfriend. I never liked him. He was permanently dirty, and his clothes looked like they had not been in the laundry for a decade. There was an awful smell always oozing from his body, and I avoided being close to him because of that smell. It was so offensive that he often insisted that I went closer to greet him. I had no clue where my mom found him or what she saw in him. He was never seen sober. He was clumsy and cleverly lazy. He was never useful to anyone. When attempting to repair a broken door handle, he made me carry everything while he talked and praised himself. One day, he collected money from my mom to buy things to repair a window. He came back with a big sandwich bag for himself with a two-liter soda and a bottle of gin. He finished his meal, the soda, and the entire bottle of gin. I don't know how he did that. He slept for the rest of the afternoon. My mom came back and cried all night.

Apart from the alcohol, another gift my mother's boyfriend had was farting. Sometimes before my mother got back from work, he would fart silently. If the smell was awful, he looked at me. "Why are you looking at me?" He laughed. Next, he mimicked the same blast with his mouth and laughed. He was nasty. He came one evening drunk as usual and started abusing my mom. He hit her hard and pushed her down on the floor. She was crying. I took one of his liquor bottles and broke it on his head. I never saw him again. I was taken by police and sent to a juvenile detention center. I hated studying, and school was not for me. I did whatever I liked, and it felt cool to do that. Later in life, I went to jail for stealing money and for drugs. After my first parole, I tried to work. I could not wait every two weeks to be paid. I got involved in selling drugs again and spent the money as quickly as it came. It was a good feeling to have money, be in charge, and buy whatever I wanted.

I was in jail every day dreaming of a beautiful home, a beautiful wife, and beautiful family. For years, I fantasized about my wedding. I was going to have an outdoor wedding in a rose garden standing side by side with my beautiful bride. She would be dressed in her wedding gown with the train sweeping the ground while I wore my white suit and black bow tie. I dreamt we would go to the Caribbean for our honeymoon. I would wake up with waiters serving us fruit. And here I am, feeling this way and languishing in this hospital, dying of cancer. I am still chained without freedom. [*He started to cry.*] I still dream about doing these things. The rest of the world is able to do them.

Many preachers told me I was made in the image of God. Was I made Friday evening when God was tired? I get it that I was an accident, that I have done so many bad things. I messed up, and I feel God is punishing me with this cancer of the liver. I caused it to myself by smoking cigarettes.

I was worn out after listening to all the things this prisoner hospitalized with cancer had to say. He had failed to live yesterday, and he was uncertain about tomorrow. I heard the sorrow of the abysmal emptiness in his heart, his struggles, and his shame. He was craving the father he never had. He was never able to feel a father's love. He longed to be accepted and loved as a human being. I felt his sense of worthlessness and his grief for failed and missed opportunities. He said he abhorred education. Did he ever have the opportunity to receive the type of education that starts at home? His life had been sealed from the beginning in this never-ending cycle of crime, poverty, and violence. This lifestyle was his daily routine and all he had ever known.

I sat there, and my heart was filled with agony for this young man. He had been carrying that cross, his shame and worthlessness, for years. He had made poor choices and had lived with the painful consequences of those choices all his life. I felt sorry for him as the world had labeled him a criminal, and he had been condemned long before he committed and was convicted of his first crime. Could he ever have a life outside of that identity? Is this how he will always be perceived—as an ex-convict? The daily things I took for granted like my family, my dad's presence, food on the table, being able to play with other children without fearing for our safety, going to church, and school were things he never had.

I held his hands and prayed with him. I prayed that God would touch his heart and heal his pain and brokenness by giving him a new heart and spirit. I felt only God could heal, restore, and welcome him to the original blessedness of the father. "Be strong and bold; have no fear or dread of them, because it is the Lord your God who goes with you; he will not fail you or forsake you" (Deuteronomy 31:6). Teaching or telling him about the promises of God as the Father would have been a waste of time when he had never felt a father's love. "Like a shepherd he feeds his flock; in his arms he gathers the lambs, carrying them in his bosom and leading the ewes with care" (Isaiah 40:10–17). I prayed that our Lord Jesus would carry him in the palm of His hands and speak to him.

We are all in need of God's grace because of our brokenness. God wondrously created us and even more wondrously restored us to grace. Every human being is created in God's image and likeness. However, when Adam and Eve fell from grace in the Garden of Eden, the door to the garden was closed. Humanity was cast out from paradise for disobeying God. We all have sinned and fallen short of the glory of God, as Saint Paul reminds us. The human body without the grace of God has an inclination for sin, greed, survival, selfishness, and egoism. Grace changes everything for us and allows us to accept love and share that love with others. All God is asking us is to trust

Him in every situation. "Have I not commanded you? Be strong and of good courage; do not be afraid, nor be dismayed, for the Lord your God is with you wherever you go" (Joshua 1:9). We are invited to be like children who put their trust in their parents to provide and care for them. God has absolute authority and the power to take care of us. When everything fails, Jesus is still there with us. Jesus wants us to place our trust in Him. We should never make the mistake of placing our trust in humans above God. Unlike humans, God is incapable of disappointing us regardless of circumstance. "This is what the Lord says: Cursed is the one who trusts in man, who draws strength from mere flesh and whose heart turns away from the Lord" (Jeremiah 17:5). God wants us to put all our trust in Him.

The happiness this young man sought was never going to be found in a life of crime or doing evil. His hunger to live and protect himself and those he loved would never be satisfied. It would be easy for him and others to assume that he deserved his current circumstance. The victims of the crimes he committed after learning of his illness would be tempted to feel that "it serves him right." This is a dangerous attitude, and it is devoid of grace. No one deserves an illness or disease. Jesus taught us to pray for our enemy and for those who persecute us. Conversely, many good people who do amazing things for humanity suffer disease. We are not entitled; neither are we guaranteed a good life just because we are good.

This prisoner still had the need to find the fullness of life. He lived out all his hopes and dreams through his imagination. I prayed for him that he would open his heart to be filled with the gifts of the Holy Spirit. Our hearts are either filled with God's grace or with the meaningless clutter that makes us miserable. The Spirit guides every human heart to live a good life. We have to open our hearts to the Holy Spirit to experience that grace. If we are not guided to encounter the Spirit, we will live selfish and self-gratifying lives, which will inevitably lead to emptiness and disillusion. "I have seen all the things that are done under the sun; all of them are meaningless, a chasing after the wind" (Ecclesiastes 1:14).

A Culture of Limitation

This prisoner at the hospital felt that from the moment he was born, his fate had been sealed. He continued the cycle of violence and disregard for others that was familiar to him. I felt that in light of his current circumstances, he had begun questioning things and seeking answers. He begun to search for his own inner voice and for meaning in life. We cannot assume that he was irredeemably lost or fundamentally flawed. However, could he love, care for others, and show appreciation like every other human being in spite of the life he had led? Who was to blame for his narrative? Was it his family, society at large, God, or himself?

This prisoner had subscribed to the idea that "I am the bad guy, and everyone else is good." Jesus says to the young man who ran up to Him and asked him, "Good teacher, what must I do to inherit eternal life?" "Why do you call me good? No one is good but God alone" (Mark 10:17). Paul, in defense of universally shared limitations, sinfulness, and brokenness of humanity, says, "All have sinned and fallen short of the glory of God" (Romans 3:23). We are all broken, and no one's brokenness is better than the other. That is why we are all in need of God's grace. The struggle to do and be good will not be over until we die. Our inner battle between good and bad is real. We all seek and cry out for God's grace and for redemption. I am not better than you; neither are you better than me. We join one another in daily prayer asking for God's grace to help us be better. We will not achieve that state of perfection until we meet God in heaven.

The environment has a powerful influence in the way we grow up and live our lives. A seed planted on fertile soil is expected to grow better than one planted in a dry desert. What makes a difference in life is our individual ability to reclaim our own voices regardless of circumstance. We have a responsibility to write our stories instead of allowing others to tell our narrative. It is not about the space but our ability to be receptive to grace whenever it comes. I feel that our sinful habits do keep us in chains, and they make us miserable here on earth. We don't even have to wait till death to experience the consequences of sin. We can start feeling them right here on earth as we live empty lives, feeling hollow inside. It creates an abyss in our hearts, and nothing ever satisfies us. Saint Paul decried, "We know that the law is spiritual; but I am unspiritual, sold as a slave to sin. I do not understand what I do. For what I want to do I do not do, but what I hate I do. And if I do what I do not want to do, I agree that the law is good. As it is, it is no longer I myself who do it, but it is sin living in me." In this passage, Paul acknowledges the struggle we all face. The following verses explain it in further detail:

> So I find this law at work: Although I want to do good, evil is right there with me. For in my inner being I delight in God's law; but I see another law at work in me, waging war against the law of my mind and making me a prisoner of the law of sin at work within me. What a wretched man I am! Who will rescue me from this body that is subject to death? Thanks be to God, who delivers me through Jesus Christ our Lord. (Romans 7:14–25)

We could easily give up on trying to be better recycling the narrative that we are helpless. Hence, we continue to hand over systemic injustice and poverty from generation to generation by reclining on this storyline of powerlessness. Honestly, to break away from a dysfunctional family is never easy. However, it is important that we do not continue to settle for the idea that it is impossible to change or procure a better life for ourselves. Evil is not our prima facie identity as humans. Seeds were sown in our lives, and the devil scattered weeds as the parable of the farmer reads, "While everyone was asleep, his enemy came and sowed tares among the wheat, and went away" (Matthew 13:25). The feeling of not being good enough is planted by the enemy, who is ever lurking and ready to disorient and misdirect us. These bad seeds try to overgrow any positive outlook we may have and obliviates any hope for a good life, thus denying our inherent ab initio goodness. Bad seeds, like bad influences, blind us to God's blessings. The Holy Spirit helps us tap into grace as it is bestowed upon us. "Blessed is the one who perseveres under trial because, having stood the test, that person will receive the crown of life that the Lord has promised to those who love him" (James 1:12).

God transcends the limits of our human nature by offering us grace. This grace allows us to return to God as illustrated by the story of the prodigal son. We cannot justify sin by saying, "God made me do it." Sin, in all its forms (selfishness, greed, gossip, murder, and violence), are primarily caused by our very arrogance. It is a feeling of entitlement that allows us to do whatever we feel like whenever we feel like it.

Every child has a dad. People may not like their dad or may never have met him. We are still his fruit. We don't choose who our biological fathers are. What we do control is our power to shut down the negativity of our culture. We must try to avoid the lethal bite of the snake and its numbing effect on our belief in the abundance of God's grace. We need to stand up to those who make us feel unworthy. Should we encounter those who call us unworthy, we need to let them see in us the abundance of God's blessings. For those who feel educated and that others are ignorant, God bless you. God has a plan for each one of us. No one can destroy us if we are not open to listen to their negativity. Their judgment should not impact us as only God knows who we really are and why we do what we do. The prisoner at the hospital felt unworthy because of his choices and the labels that society had given him. The reality was that he was indeed in jail, but not beyond redemption. His jail experience was only part of his story. He was not completely lost. He still had an enormous sense of love and duty for his mother, who had not aborted or abandoned him. This prisoner needed to focus on the good in him and allow God's grace to envelope him during his time of suffering. We need to strive to find our own purpose and define our destiny.

Invitation to Charity

Everyone has value and can contribute to the well-being of others. As a leaking vessel can be used as a flower pot, each one of us plays a role. Someone who is ninety-nine years old is a gift, particularly to their family, but also to those whose lives they touched while in service to humanity. There is a tendency in this world to compartmentalize things and put them in a box. People place their own expectations on others, and when those expectations are not met, the ugly labels start. It is through God's grace that we are able to stand and not be defined by those labels.

I remember visiting a man in the neuroscience unit. He had some type of memory loss. He was agitated during our first encounter, and I was not quite certain I should go back. However, I did visit him again. He complained and was panicking because the doctor had recommended that his driving license be taken away. I intentionally sat with him and allowed him to work through his feelings as he struggled to accept his new reality. Our conversation seemed endless, but I left fulfilled knowing that in that moment, he needed a friend and companion. I also reminded him that giving up his driver's license for the safety of others is an act of love and kindness not because he is a burden. That act requires courage. He called out to me and recalled most of my conversations with him:

> I am at this hospital in pain and gripped by fear for the uncertainties ahead of me. I am losing my memory. It was very distressing at first. I tried to make sense of all of this, but I couldn't. I really appreciate the gifts you gave to me. Now I can say that I have received the gift of peace without really knowing how or understanding why. My experience lying in this hospital bed was one of learning to trust God beyond my circumstances, to see the beauty in the shadows of life and accept it as is. I believe God will see me through even when I don't know how. There is a newness and renewed meaning for my life. Accepting love and being cared for was not a sign of my becoming old and weak. I saw that no matter what is going on, God has always stood by me, even when I did

not see Him. He was the source of my life, and I
am in His hands to nourish and sustain me.

One day, I got a short note from the man saying, "Thank you
so much. You brought so much comfort to me. You projected such
a profound aura of comfort and calm that I felt safe talking to you. I
felt listened to and not judged. I rattled through all my fears, worries,
and anxieties, and you stood there and paid attention. Thank you so
much." This is a great testimony from the man. I couldn't reach him
to say thank *you* so much. It was uplifting for me to see that even in
the midst of uncertainty and the stress of life, there is a glimpse of
grace. Grace is always available if we are open to find it in unfamiliar
places and circumstances. I had merely reminded this man of the fact
that he had served others and that perhaps it was time to give himself grace to accept love. He understood that it was not a matter of
becoming dependent but an opportunity to give grace to those who
wanted to minister to him.

Our story is not yet over. We are alive to testify to the goodness
of God. I have reminded the prisoner and everybody who needed
to hear it that God is always with us and that our stories are not
over yet. I reminded them that every day on this earth is a day to
bless someone. The prisoner was given an opportunity to rewrite his
story by doing simple things even in prison. It is not just about the
past. What people remember is how touched they were even by a
small gesture. He had a choice about how his fellow inmates would
remember him. He had the power to affect the guards with whom
he came in contact. What a marvelous thing it would be if those
guards were to go home and tell their families what a blessing he had
become. God has given us the pen to write our own stories. It is up
to us to grab the pen and write our own story or allow the enemy to
write it for us. It is also up to us to be the blessing that others will
write about when narrating their own stories.

As generous distributors of God's manifold grace,
put your gifts at the service of one another, each
in the measure he has received. The one who

speaks is to deliver God's message. The one who serves is to do it with the strength provided by God. Thus, in all of you God is to be glorified through Jesus Christ. (1 Peter 4:10–11)

In the parable of the lost sheep, the shepherd goes in search of the one and leaves the ninety-nine. God the Father is searching for us. We remember the story of Joseph the dreamer. He was sold as a slave by his brothers and ended up in Egypt. They did not know God's plan, and they felt they had rid themselves of him. After many years had passed, they went to Egypt; and unbeknownst to them, they would end up at Joseph's mercy. They pleaded for forgiveness and even asked to be accepted as slaves. Joseph, in his wisdom, said, "Don't be afraid. Am I in the place of God? You intended to harm me, but God intended it for good to accomplish what is now being done, the saving of many lives" (Genesis 50:19–20). God's plan had prevailed. When it comes to healing, we all have a role to play in offering support to others especially in the most vulnerable time of their lives when they feel empty and abandoned. We will now look at the fact that we all share in this ministry of compassion. We are called to offer support to one another daily.

Part V

THE GLORY

"And the Word became flesh, and dwelt among us, and we saw His glory, glory as of the only begotten from the Father, full of grace and truth" (John 1:14).

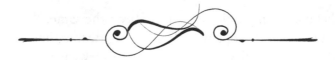

The Ascent to Acceptance

In the summer of 2016, I had the incredible experience of going hiking to Jasper National Park with students from Holy Cross High School, Saskatoon, Canada. We prepared for this trip by walking for almost two hours, climbing stairs, hills, and those who could not cope dropped out. I still remember my surprise looking at the list of items we were required to carry on a hiking trip. We carried plenty of water, things to eat, rain gear, sanitary tissues, and things for safety. We walked for hours and hours, journeying through the rocks, hills, and crossing streams before getting to the top of the mountain.

Laboriously gasping for air as we got to the mountaintop, seeing and touching the ice on the glacier, feeling the crisp air, hearing the wind chiming in a melodious rhythm, and penetrating the clouds—was all mystical and magical to me. The hardship of climbing to get to the top of the mountain was absolutely worth it. I felt that incredible delight in my heart getting to more than twelve thousand feet elevation. I was in the presence of something larger than I could comprehend. It was like Saint Peter's experience during the Transfiguration when Jesus appeared to the three disciples in radiant beauty on the mountain, and Peter said, "Lord it is good for us to be here. Let us build three tents" (Matthew 17:1–9).

Climbing to the peak of the mountain was tough. Experiencing the majesty of the mountaintop was glorious and beautiful. I had always seen pictures and watched movies of glaciers and was amazed by their serenity and beauty. The lakes around those mountains were crystal clear and unimaginably beautiful. Climbing the mountains to experience that for myself was priceless. I would not trade the experience of walking through rough tracks and stones to get to the top of the mountain for anything, not even for being dropped off at the top with a helicopter. It would never have been the same. When climbing mountains, there are always frightening distractions. For me, as I looked down the valley, the depth of the valley gave me pause, and I felt dizzy and thought I was going to fall. I avoided the temptation to check out any other cliffs after that experience.

We can equate my experience of climbing Mount Columbia in Jasper National park with how rough, treacherous, and dangerous the journey of life can be. It feels much like looking down at the valley from the hilltop and knowing there is a risk of dying. In life, we face many obstacles and challenges, and it seems easier to give up. Being sick at the hospital is one of those rough times that frightens us while on our life journey. We need grace to remain focused on this journey as we head toward our final destination. Life is rough and difficult. The experience of bliss and the crown of glory as the ultimate goal is what motivates us to endure the tough journey to the end. The sun, low altitude, dry air, the rain and the wind absolutely challenged us. They also helped us appreciate the beauty around us. We were tempted to give up, but through grace and determination, we made it to the end. We must allow the grace of God to be part of our journey. Grace helps us to turn our everyday experience of pain and sickness into glory.

Every victory comes after a fight and at a price. If the journey is easy, we cannot call it a victory. Being victorious actually means that we were involved in a battle and we won the fight. After our climb through unfriendly terrain, harsh weather, diminished oxygen due to altitude, and exhaustion, we made it to the top. I felt our effort was rewarded, and the mountain exclaimed, *Welcome, you made it. Thanks for your courage.* I raised my hands and shouted, "I made it! I am here! I did it! I conquered it!"

Acceptance Is Transformative

I met a farmer at the hospital who had been recently diagnosed with alveolitis, a disease that affected his lungs. He said he had noticed that he was having difficulty breathing, started feeling weak, and had a bad cough. For many months, he went to his family doctor and was given cough medicines to control his coughing. As he continued to have difficulty breathing, he returned and was placed on antibiotics until it became obvious that something was really wrong. He was referred to Hershey Hospital, and they found out he had this disease. He shared how he found peace trusting God:

> I am a Christian and said my daily prayers. Whenever I faced a difficulty that I couldn't solve, I prayed for God's help, and He was always there for me. I learned to trust Him in every situation. I was a high school football coach for many years. I depended on God during my coaching days, and He helped me trust Him more. As a farmer, I went through a lot of losses and gains; God was there with me. I could never have gone through those challenges and survive without the grace of God. In all adversities, God has been gracious to me and pulled me through. I know He will also pull me through this.

Time in the hospital can connect us to the sacredness of our being, or it can make us sad and fragmented. Suffering in life is sacred because it prepares us to behold the glory being revealed in God. Crosses and happiness are neighbors of the human condition. Sometimes we feel terrific and excited about things around us, and other times we are downcast. We may be genuinely concerned about the uncertainty of the future. When the storms of life appear, how we carry the heavy weight on our shoulder as we swim across the river is important. The problem is when we allow suffering and grace to exist in opposition to each other instead of understanding that suffering sheds light into the glory being revealed. As suffering, sickness, hunger, and death are part of our human existence; likewise, happiness, joy, and peace are paramount to revealing glory.

God prepares us for a special mission on a daily basis. We are called upon to journey with Him and wait patiently for our own time. Precious metals like gold and diamonds are not found on the surface of the earth. We have to dig to find them. Sometimes we break through ice, mud, rocks, and have to remove other unwanted material until it is found. When we find it, it is a source of an abundance of wealth. Like a woman who, after labor, smiles and does not remember the pains she went through, our joy will be complete. When God lifts us out of suffering and positions us where He wants us, the price we paid will be forgotten. We are called to surrender to God. We should listen and trust Him because He is faithful. He never disappointed anyone who put their trust in Him, and God will not do that to His children. For the Lord who started the good work in you will bring it to completion.

When sick, we come to the hospital to be healed through the hands of the doctors, nurses, and others in the health ministry. This healing of our physical body happens quicker when we find grace in our suffering. This moment of grace heals our stress and anxiety and prepares us to receive physical healing from the ailment. I thank God for the testimonies of healing happening daily. We do not often hear about those blessings and graces. These graces do happen. We do not often see the hand of God in it all, and at times feel we are entitled to it. I stood in admiration listening to this farmer in his struggle, pain, fear, faith, and the strength of the spirit being revealed in his sickness. Finding grace, beauty, and peace in the midst of fear restores us to wholeness. This restoration is a gift of grace. Beyond the fear and pain, we find peace that brings comfort to us. This gift of peace despite our condition brings us and our loved ones the kind of healing that far surpasses our physical condition.

The mountain was rough and tough, but so is carrying our crosses with joy and enthusiasm because of the pain we endure. We need grace to overcome the pain and suffering we face. These could be caused by sickness, poverty, humiliation, loneliness, rejection, and abandonment, among others. The grace to overcome any of these comes through our openness to God's gift of grace. Without the grace of God, the burdens of life are so stressful that life becomes a living hell. We have to understand that opening our hearts to grace does not lessen the weight of the cross. We experience some good and some bad days. We do not always receive compliments from those we make sacrifices for, and neither do we expect that.

Unfortunately, a little appreciation would be helpful in encouraging us. We are often afraid to show our deepest emotions of dissatisfaction and unhappiness when not appreciated. We should not allow the suffering we go through to distract us from trusting and hoping in God. Being guided by the grace of God is pertinent for our healing and experience of mercy.

> Not only that, but we must rejoice in our suffering, knowing that suffering produces endurance, and endurance produces character, and character produces hope, and hope does not put us to shame, because God's love has been poured into our hearts through the Holy Spirit who has been given to us. (Romans 5:3–5)

This openness to acceptance is an incarnational experience which gives meaning and purpose to our suffering, which would otherwise render us helpless and open to accepting meaninglessness.

Acceptance Is Incarnational

To find meaning in times of suffering is an invitation to grace. It is an incarnational journey of rebirth in which we are open to not passively accept suffering and its pain. We are reborn because of it; we change either in a transformative way, or we are destroyed by despondency. In the darkness of the womb, we experienced living under the protection and providence of our mother. For nine months, we were totally dependent on our mother's nourishment even while our eyes were closed. It is in the dark that we learn total dependence. In the womb, we were never afraid; we were in a state of grace and totally dependent on our mother and oblivious to what was happening around us. We never worried about what tomorrow would bring. We were living in the dark but filled with grace.

This experience with darkness allows for the manifestation of the gift of grace when we feel lost and we live in despair and hopelessness. The incarnational experience enables us to transform inexplicable suffering into something worthwhile. Our pain has meaning. Instead of accepting despair, we triumph over it and experience a newness of sorts. Our new way of life becomes the new normal, and we are at peace. We give purpose and find personal fulfilment in our brokenness.

I visited a patient who was sixteen when she first started her battle with cancer. While her friends were joyfully getting their driver's licenses, she was at the hospital fighting for her life and receiving chemotherapy. She said she had learned what was important in life at that tender age. She had a very positive attitude. She said something like, "With everything I have been through in life, I cannot but appreciate God's blessings. It is difficult to hear the groans of the patient next door, and sleep is at a premium. I know that it is not easy for him. My nurse told me she is working with a nursing student, and I asked her to bring her so she can learn how to draw blood and hook my IV. If I can help someone learn how to reach out to others and be a better nurse, it would be a good enough reason for me to be at the hospital now."

This positive attitude blew my mind. I saw that she was able to experience a rebirth through the suffering that she was enduring. Like a child in the darkness of the mother's womb, totally dependent for nourishment and life, God wants us to depend on him. "I depend on God alone; I put my hope in him. He alone protects and saves me; he is my defender, and I shall never be defeated. My salvation and honor depend on God; he is my strong protector; he is my shelter" (Psalm 62:5–7).

The womb is empty, dark, and yet expandable. If the womb were not expandable, if it were occupied by something else, we would not have space to grow, mature, and be born. Unless we open our hearts and embrace God's abundant grace, we will never find the beauty in our darkest moments. God pours His grace unto us, but we have to be open to be filled by it. When we are not open to God's grace, many other things fill our grace-destined spaces. We become filled with the junk that surrounds us every day. We live our lives in grace and are surrounded by darkness. We are not able to see the giver of life around us if we do not allow ourselves to be nourished by God. Without God's gift of grace, we cannot enter the kingdom of beauty, peace, serenity that is silently dwelling in darkness. That is the experience of heaven, "Thy kingdom come."

This mystical image of the light of grace pouring in to heal our brokenness was clearly depicted in Rubem Alves's book *Transparencies of Eternity*:

> Beauty is a volatile entity—it touches the skin and quickly vanishes. The name of God is like that: a great, huge space that houses all the beauty of the universe. If the glass were not empty, we wouldn't be able to fill it to drink from it. If the mouth were not empty, we wouldn't be able to eat fruit. If the womb were not empty, life wouldn't grow in it. If the sky were not empty, birds, clouds and kites wouldn't be able to fly.

As with a mother's womb, the fragility of life, emptiness, darkness, serenity, and beauty are all intertwined. They all fill creation and are part of the natural order of the human existential family. We couldn't run away from them in this fallen world. In this same vein, we cannot avoid being affected by what our mothers eat while carrying us in the womb. That is all part of the interconnectedness that forms our beings. These realities are an integral part of who we are. Unfortunately, when we continuously partake in the journey of human life, we create room for darkness. We judge in the absence of grace. The brokenness, hurt, disappointment, loneliness, failure, and shame we go through in life are part of what makes us who we are. They are all part of us just as the food and nutrients that form our entire being in the womb.

The trials people go through in life could be terrifying. Patients feel abandoned, lonely, and hopelessly lost in the dark. Jesus was buried and left to decay in the tomb after his death. The Jewish authorities expected that after the monstrous abuse Jesus had endured, his body would decompose fast. Soldiers sealed the tomb with heavy stones so the smell of decay would not offend the community. He was left alone while everyone went back to the community to tell His story, how He suffered, and how He died. They narrated how His heart was pierced to make sure he was dead. They shared how he was given vinegar instead of water and the crown of thorns that tortured him till He died. Despite what everyone else was saying about Jesus's demise, Jesus changed the narrative of the story. He replaced the putrid smell of the tomb with the fragrance of love and compassion from His mother, Mary, who was full of grace. His body did not experience corruption or decay. While the women were hoping to find who could help them roll away the stone, Jesus had already moved it.

The women who had gone to the tomb to anoint His body with perfume were in shock. His body was no longer in the tomb, and there were no traces of a decomposing body. The other disciples could not find His body either. However, the empty tomb was no longer empty. There had been a new birth. Darkness could no longer dwell in the empty tomb; the light of Jesus shone forever. Jesus's death and the darkness of the empty tomb represent the fullness of grace and a new life and faith in Christ. "The disciples remembered that he told them that he would rise from the dead after three days" (John 2:22).

At the resurrection, Jesus changed the narrative of the story of His burial in the tomb. His disciples had confirmation of the resurrection through the empty tomb. No one saw Him rise. He did not allow any human the privilege of seeing the drama of the rock that sealed the tomb rolling backward. He did not make a show of His coming out of the tomb with the bright light of His resurrection dispelling the darkness of the tomb. He gave them permission to see Him after the resurrection. He sent them into the world to be witnesses to a resurrection that they had not watched. They told the story of the drama they did not see unfold. Some of His disciples died because of their faith in the incredible power of the resurrection.

The empty tomb where Jesus was buried became a fountain of faith and hope for the disciples. He took all our sins and afflictions with Him and nailed them to the cross. It was the old nature we inherited from Adam that He took with Him. As He died on the cross, He said, "It is finished." He buried this Adamic body in the tomb, and with it was our sinful nature. In the Easter resurrection, He transformed our natural body and made us His children by adoption. We are all new creations, as Saint Paul says. Old things have passed away, and all things have become new. It is this grace of new life in Christ that we experience as He shares in our suffering. He buried our suffering in the tomb so that as we place our trust in Him, no power of evil will ever touch us. Without His grace, nothing would ever satisfy us in that emptiness. Nothing dispels the darkness in the empty tomb if we don't experience the transformative power of Jesus, who is the resurrection and life.

It gave them new energy to move on in life and be witnesses to the resurrection even to the point of dying for their faith. Without connecting to the fountain of grace from the empty tomb, our lives would be empty when facing suffering. The grace of God is what changes our narrative in times of suffering so that the emptiness we experience can be transformed by grace.

The hospital makes us feel empty. We are scared because it is like being in the dark. It brings us into that awareness of our humanity, powerlessness, and lack of control over the things around us. There is no other time we are more exposed to this vulnerability than when we are at the hospital. Sickness exposes us to weakness and dependability. We become fragile, volatile, and awfully powerless. It exposes us to danger as the emptiness we experience could be readily filled by fear and anxiety. With Jesus, the tomb is not empty. In the same vein, with Jesus at the hospital, the bed would not be empty. He is with us in that emptiness with His glorified body.

Acceptance Is Overcoming Meaninglessness

Life is filled with ups and downs. No matter how good we may feel life is, once in a while, we do experience excruciating suffering that is undoubtedly overwhelming to say the least. How we relate or handle the situation is clearly what makes the difference. Suffering could be a motivation to change, get insight, which will provide meaningfulness. Suffering may also lead to psychological trauma if we can't find purpose, fulfilment, or meaning to our life because of our condition. Overcoming our suffering—be it physical, psychological, social, or spiritual—is only possible if the experience is transformative. What gives suffering this meaning is when we see it as life-changing, something for a greater cause and something we do because of higher love. Without this motivation, we could easily become despondent and enter into the oblivion of meaninglessness.

There have been times while working at the hospital when I have felt overcome by my prejudices and judgement. However, every day I learn that it is something I have to improve on. I thought that after many years serving God, being with the sick, praying with them, and sharing in their pain, I would be comfortable doing what I do. But it is becoming clearer to me that learning is something I have to do daily. It is an uphill battle that I never win.

A young woman gave a long diatribe which included fancy medical words to describe her ailment. She was in her early thirties. She had been going through chemotherapy and radiation treatments for a year since her diagnosis, but she was getting worse. Based on what she had said, I understood it was cancer and deliberately avoided asking what type. Her youth was what pained me the most. She had young kids, and all her worries were centered around who would take care of her kids. During this first visit, I was extremely touched by her story and lamentations. She said she had stage four cancer and was told she only had few days, weeks, or months to live.

She looked healthy in spite of her dire diagnosis. She talked and talked while I listened. I do not understand why something like this should ever happen to anyone. She lamented that she would not be there to see her children grow up. She would not be attending their graduations and weddings. As I listened to her, my heart sunk watching her in tears, especially while expressing her anguish at not being able to see her children grow or having them be raised by "another woman," as she put it. The only comfort I found was the knowledge that in our brokenness, Jesus was with us. She requested I visit her again, which I promised to do.

I went the next day to see her, and she said she was tired. A few days later, I got a request for a priest's visit and I went. We chatted briefly and she said she was tired so I left. I saw her request and decided to check on her. She thanked me for visiting, but she was indisposed that day. After these multiple experiences, my brain started raising red flags. *Why do I have to check on her again? Why do I care for her? If she is spiritually dehydrated, she has to seek for water for herself. It is not my responsibility to go around looking to quench people's thirst.* That was my inner struggle until I got a call to administer her last rites.

It was embarrassing for me because I kept telling myself that I had allowed my prejudice to override my better judgement. Maybe she had been struggling, hurting, broken, and did not even know how to face God and her pain. For her, I am God's representative, and maybe she did not know what to do. But what was I supposed to do? Was I to beg to see her? Was I to walk into the room every time and be told I was not welcome? How many times should I walk into a room before I realize I am becoming a nuisance instead of being of help? That was my struggle, and I know I had given up on making any effort to check in on her again.

As I walked into her room for the Last Rites, I was surprised to see her alert and talking. She said, "Father, thanks for coming. I am happy you are here. I was so scared of dying. I was in a coma, and I was terrified with all the things I saw. I saw so many disfigured faces looking at me, and I was afraid. I tried to talk to my brother. He could not even hear me. I felt alone and abandoned. If dying is what I saw, there is no way I want to die. I know everything happens for a reason. Things happen because God wants. I wonder why God is letting me go through all this suffering. I was never a bad person. I was not really mean, and I am not saying I was ever perfect. I don't think I deserve to go through all the things I am facing."

Her sister by her side said to her, "You should remember that all suffering happens for a reason. We may not understand it, but God knows why those things happen. We are made to go through suffering so we can experience the glory of God."

She interrupted her, saying, "I don't want you to say that. I have said it again and again. No one is listening to me or seems to understand what I am going through. Let Father speak and answer my question. He is the only one I felt paid attention to what I was trying to say. So don't speak."

I said the her, "I know it is not easy to face the type of suffering that you are experiencing now. It is distressing. Unfortunately, the easy answers we were taught to offer support do not help in these situations. Sometimes they hurt us more instead of comforting and healing our wounds. So there is nothing wrong with accepting that we do not have answers but that we are searching for meaning. I know that saints' quotes and Hallmark-style ready-made phrases may not always be of help. So I feel we can agree that you have every right to say you are angry with God."

I remember pondering, *In this sacred space of suffering and fear of hopelessness, what do I tell her? What words could ever bring consolation to her?* I was surprised when the next question came.

"Father, if you were dying, what would you do? If you were like me, not knowing how long you had to live, hours, days, weeks or months, what would you do?"

I was in shock. Where to start? What should I say? It was such a personal and direct question that there was no avoiding it.

"I did not anticipate that question. I didn't even know where to start to answer. However, I will say that if I had a few days to live, I would invite my family for blessings. I would ask them to pray for me too. I would reconcile with God, those I offended, and those who offended me. I would invite God into my heart and make peace. If anything happened, I would not want to have to say, 'Had I known.' Getting myself ready would require much grace. If I had time, I would like to travel and enjoy my time."

Then she continued, "I was not a bad person. I did my best to live a decent life and played by the rules. This sickness sucks. This is not what I would wish even to my worst enemy. It is difficult for me to face death. I was really hoping and praying. It is painful to see my dreams shattered, to lie in this hospital for months without any hope of recovering. So why hope when I know there is nothing to hope for? No dream to be fulfilled and all the wonderful things I was hoping to do in life were destroyed in the blink of an eye. I prayed. I tried to bargain with God and said, 'Please allow me to live, and I will dedicate my life to doing good.' In the end, this is the outcome. It is terrible to hope for good things because it is frustrating when you get negative results. This cancer has changed everything for me. I dared to hope, and now that hope has vanished."

I then said to her, "So if you were to reconcile with yourself, others, and God, where would you start?"

"I think I would start by going to confession. But I have not done that for years. I went to a Catholic school for twelve years. I would always speak to God directly. And besides, you are my friend. There is no way I will start telling my sins to you. I have a question, though. Do people really tell the truth while confessing to a priest? Do they actually confess everything they did? We used to make a list when it was our turn or just repeat the last ones for which the priest had given us the least penance."

That made me laugh. "Hard to imagine that everyone felt that confession was but a list of sins read to the priests. Their intention was good, but some did not really understand the abundance of grace that dwells in the confessional. We go to confession to heal the inner wounds we have in our hearts. The priest, who at that moment is standing as Christ, prays with us for forgiveness. He is our companion in moments of brokenness. I am not there to judge you, and there is nothing you are going to say that would diminish the respect I have for you. Confession is a time we spend asking God to heal our brokenness, our heart, guilt, shame, and pain. It is the moment we face our inadequacies without shame and overcome our pride with humility to avoid the humiliation of sin. It is a healing sacrament in which we surrender our brokenness at the feet of the cross. It is that special time when we open our hearts to receive the mercy of God in abundance. It goes beyond the priest as we ask for prayers, and the priest leads us in that prayerful moment." No sooner had I said this, she asked to have her confession heard, and she received communion.

"Father, thanks. You won't believe how much better I feel. It is as if a heavy load has been lifted off my shoulders. I am going to call my mom and tell her I went to confession. She is not going to believe that I actually asked to do it. She will be in shock when she hears that I received communion again. Thanks so much for this moment."

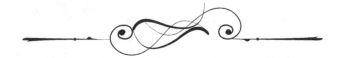

Experiencing "Supersonic Love"

In 2017, I had the opportunity to visit my family in Nigeria. I had not seen them for some years. I planned to surprise my mother with this visit aided by my friends and siblings. When I arrived, everyone in the compound welcomed me, screaming in elation. My mother could not stop screaming and hugging me. She didn't even remember that her feet had been hurting as she jumped up to embrace me. She tried to lift me up but couldn't. She hugged, kissed, and exclaimed in my dialect, "Welcome, welcome, and welcome from your journey." She embraced me again and held me tighter as if trying to prevent me from running away. There was a look of amazement as she exclaimed, "Are you really here? This is such a pleasant surprise." I saw the joyful confusion on her face, and I just laughed. She was overwhelmed with joy and started singing and praising God because I had arrived safely.

That's what I call a dose of supersonic love. It is an unexpected favor characterized by massive amounts of joy and love that cloud any feeling of pain or discomfort. We are also able to experience a supersonic type of love when we become aware of God's grace and love during times of dire need. We are inexplicably able to experience the intoxicating love that is revealed to us by God's grace in those times when darkness abounds and hope is not even a word that we recognize. Those around us would fail to understand why our hearts are filled with joy. This epiphany is God's gift of His supersonic love for us. It gives new meaning and purpose to our lives. With this new light, we marvel at God's awesomeness because we become more aware of His presence even when we thought ourselves alone and abandoned.

Suffering has a way to make us experience darkness. It blinds us to the beauty and awesomeness of things around us and eclipses the experience of joy and excitement we long for. We often wonder, when will this be over? Focusing on the glory that is being revealed to us in our suffering helps us along the journey. That is the grace God gives to us.

For many patients, the experience of being at the hospital serves as a time of encountering the epiphany of God's grace. Many people experience this surprising perspective and peace because God revealed His presence right by their bedsides at the hospital. Setting foot at the hospital can reveal to us the gift of the life we have. Spending time at the hospital in whatever capacity—be it as a patient, family member, or friend—can help us appreciate how finite our lives really are. It could serve as a reminder that we should value our time. It could be that time when we lose our blindfold to see the revelation of God's beauty in the world. When that happens, it is the greatest gift. God continues to reveal His love to us in surprising ways every day. He draws us closer to Himself so that we may see the beauty and the healing taking place around us. And above all, we must be open and appreciate those moments when God showers us with His supersonic love.

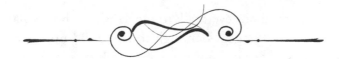

Revelation of God's Presence

Every life is conceived in the womb of a woman. Even when the woman donates her egg, life happens because she opened herself up to receiving the gift of the male sperm. This is when the fullness of grace is ratified. The womb is the space where our life began. Jesus was conceived in the womb of the Virgin Mary, who carried him for nine months. When Jesus died on the cross, those who killed Him thought His story was over. They were ignorant of God's plan. The Good Friday experience was just the beginning. Mary, who is full of grace, carried his body and waited for burial. The angel Gabriel said, "Hail Mary, full of grace." From the time of His holy conception and into His death, she displayed an abundance of grace.

When we know that Jesus stands by us in times of sickness and darkness, our hope is alive. We will not be afraid of darkness in the empty tomb because we know that we are never alone in that emptiness, and that is comforting. Even in our darkest moments, we can see the light of Jesus as it shines to bring us peace and comfort. When we experience suffering in the light of grace, it is like a reawakening for us. Hence, in that experience, the light of God dispels the darkness of pain, fear, and despair. It dispels confusion and brings calm into our empty tomb of disorientation and anxiety. It is in this light of grace that we will see Jesus as He stands with us to defend us in every situation we face. He is our good friend who never abandons us and is always there to suffer with us. "Though my father and mother forsake me, the Lord will receive me" (Psalm 27:10). With the conviction that Jesus is with us, we know that the tomb is never empty because we have a companion even when we are in the dark.

One day, one of the patients said to me, "I have another question. Since my cancer diagnosis, my friends have avoided me. My closest friends could not even talk to me to ask me how I was doing. Those who were courageous enough to come did not even ask me how I was doing. They did not want me to tell them what was going on. They would tell me about their dogs, the movies they watched, and all the wonderful things their kids were doing at school. Some of them talked about their new jobs, new clothes, and their vacation plans. It was useless chatter about which YouTube influencer had the highest rating and who was leading social media rankings. It was terribly depressing to listen to this meaningless chatter. They had no clue the effect that had on me. It was not that I wanted to be rude. I deliberately closed my eyes, and they thought I had fallen asleep. It hurt very much."

It was at this time that I said to her, "Keep in mind that these friends are a reflection of the culture in which we live. It is a life-style that does not like to address suffering and death. It is a culture that tries to avoid or numb pain. It is a culture that encourages fake images and Photoshop to make us look glamorous while hiding the brokenness inside. We are supposed to fight against cancer. We are never to accept aging because that is not appealing. We have to mod-ify our looks to achieve a perfect appearance. It is a world in which we are never to accept weakness and failure. We must always be on top and in charge and 'win.' To accept the perils of illness when we have fought with everything we had is tantamount to accepting defeat. It becomes a life without hope. It blinds us to seeing grace, glory, and victory only when we 'win.' It is only when things go our own way and how we expect them to go that they are good. This is the new language of the new generation that dreams of a perfect world. We have to fight the finite nature of life and the limitations that are part of our human condition."

Earth has been expected to become paradise here on earth. We are no longer in a fallen world because the world becomes infinite in that light. It is a world in which everything starts and ends in this life. There is no afterlife for which we need to be prepared. Our focus is only on this existence. The views and way of life of these friends are therefore a reflection of the mundane, vain, and frivolous aspects of this world. We swim in triviality, and we make it what matters. The hospital makes us face the reality that the most important thing in life isn't me. It is a shocking reality that many of us try to avoid or want to pretend does not exist. We want to talk about our dogs, our travels, makeup, and new reality shows, but we skirt topics as the sacredness of life. We avoid them because they remind us of the pain of our vulnerability and emptiness. We are forced to depart from that fantasy world to enter the reality of our weaknesses and limitations. As human, we cannot conquer death, aging, and dying. We cannot escape death. It is there with us.

Remember in times of suffering and difficulty, not all friends would risk standing with us. Some sing our praises only in good times. Though few, good friends willingly share in our suffering. I asked her to read the book of Sirach, "For there are friends when it suits them, but they will not be around in time of trouble. Another is a friend who turns into an enemy, and tells of the quarrel to your disgrace. Others are friends, table companions, but they cannot be found in time of affliction. When things go well, they are your other self, and lord it over your servants. If disaster comes upon you, they turn against you and hide themselves. Stay away from your enemies, and be on guard with your friends. Faithful friends are a sturdy shelter; whoever finds one finds a treasure. Faithful friends are beyond price. No amount can balance their worth. Faithful friends are life-saving medicine; those who fear God will find them." (Sirach 6:8-16) She was surprised to read that these experiences were already clearly stated in the Bible.

As we enjoy the gift of grace, we are no longer afraid to look for answers to fill our emptiness. Jesus, who is always with us, is the best answer. This revelation of the sufficiency of God's grace in times of need is satisfying. It is incredibly beautiful as we no longer experience angst about finding answers. Our hearts burst with joy when faced with the beauty of God's grace.

When we encounter Jesus in our brokenness, His love fills and heals us. "I came that you may have life, and have it more abundantly" (John 10:10). When Jesus fills us with the abundance of His blessings, our focus will cease to be on our physical pain and situation. Focusing on the physical aspect of our existence creates more anxiety, fear, and despair. When Christ Jesus is by our side, we see clearly that we will not be held captive in the tomb. The experience of darkness in the tomb is temporal because the light of Christ's resurrection will dispel the darkness of uncertainty. The tomb will cease to be a scary place. It will become a place for celebration because Jesus, who is our light, brings His light into it. The hospital will be a place to share our testimony of beauty and serenity beyond circumstance. It will become a place of communion, beauty, love, worship, trust, togetherness, exploration, elevation, solemnity, and mystery into that sacred space to bring comfort to us. "And even though my illness was a trial to you, you did not treat me with contempt or scorn. Instead, you welcomed me as if I were an angel of God, as if I were Christ Jesus himself" (Galatians 4:14).

Hidden Glory Revealed

When we look at the interconnectedness between suffering and glory, no matter the cross we have to bear, our outlook changes. The glory being revealed in suffering changes our perception and gives new meaning to our lives. It eases the pain we experience in suffering and makes it bearable. A hospitalization could be a terrible experience. When it happens, we do everything possible to get out as soon as possible. Sickness and any form of suffering can be terrifying. We are not in control of the timing or the outcome.

I was spellbound the first time I heard the story behind the song "It Is Well with My Soul." We sang this song in church a thousand times. Horatio Spafford, a lawyer, wrote this song after enduring the most tragic of experiences. He very sadly had to endure the death of his son at the tender age of two. In 1871, the Great Chicago fire destroyed the property in which he had invested. He was to travel with his family to Europe, but because of a business emergency, he stayed back and sent the family ahead of him. During their transatlantic voyage, the *Ville du Havre* ocean liner carrying his family sunk. he lost his four daughters, and only his wife survived. The wife, Anna Spafford, sent him a telegraph: "Saved alone what shall I do?" She also told him about her other friends and their children who had died. It was after that traumatic experience that he wrote "It Is Well with My Soul." At the lowest point of his life, in the midst of this traumatic and tragic experience, Spafford still found a deeper voice that cried out beyond his physical pain, "It is well with my soul." He found the grace that came from God in his brokenness to experience peace and serenity. He survived this painful tragedy by opening his heart to God, who revealed His abundance of grace to him even in his numerous losses. He encountered the glory of the love of God revealed in the cross.

Like Spafford, many people carry their crosses effortlessly without complaining. It amazes me to meet these people who are able to bear their crosses with such dignity, elegance, and joy. They may be at the hospital, in prison, or in their homes. I have great admiration and respect for so many families looking after their loved ones at home for years. Caring for family members with disabilities or mental illness and ministering to the dying at home requires special grace. There are so many families who do not have the ability to care for their loved ones at home. Each and every one of us shares in the suffering of Christ. We endure the challenges of human existence.

When we reach out to help and care for one another, we clearly exemplify the unseen power of grace. We manifest our love by being the healing hands of Jesus to our loved ones. Many of these families who are caring for their loved ones have experienced grace and turned the cross into glory. They do not see caring for their loved ones as a cross to bear. They consider it a gift and the revelation of God's glory. In that moment, the physical reality is conquered by this revealing, unquenchable fire of love. This indestructible love melts away the pain of suffering due to sickness into the abundance of God's grace. This does not mean that the suffering is no longer real; they do live with pain and struggle. The difference is their attitude toward their situation. Once they experience the grace of God, they become aware of the mystery of the hidden bliss that is bountifully present in that sacred space. This experience is the glory being revealed as Saint Peter stated, "But rejoice inasmuch as you participate in the suffering of Christ, so that you may be overjoyed when his glory is revealed" (1 Peter 4:13).

Patients carrying their crosses with grace became a source of learning for me to trust God more and more. They challenge me to accept the graces God has bestowed upon me. Many of these people still see God's glory and beauty in their difficulty, and that is what is amazing about it. I looked in awe and with trepidation at the abundance of grace flowing from these people who carry their crosses effortlessly while following Christ. They reach this level of acceptance and growth in their life journey by opening their hearts to receive God's grace. They allow that grace to pour on others to heal our world. I feel they have experienced an intimate union with Jesus in His suffering. Their struggle ceased to be problematic and turned glorious. This experience enabled them to reach spiritual illumination, and they do not feel alone. "But the Lord stood at my side and gave me strength" (2 Timothy 4:17). They no longer see it as suffering but as their share in the abundance of grace. The immensity of this grace pours continuously from the side of the Lamb slain on the cross. This higher relationship with the Divine in our human weakness conquers suffering and transcends physical conditions. It elevates our woes to the presence of the Lamb in an eschatological and transcendent union where they become purified. "And behold, I am coming quickly, and my reward is with Me, to give to every one according to his work" (Revelation 22:12).

We are in a world where things happen to those who are good and those who are bad. No human being is immune from the illnesses and diseases facing the world. The patient is not a victim of sickness but is broken to experience the Transfiguration in Christ Jesus. They enter paradise for themselves not in death but in a new living experience where they find grace exactly as and where they are in life. Their experiences transcend the pain and fear of their conditions, and they faithfully stand to reclaim a new science. This science is the mystery of grace. It is our petition, hunger, and desire to find grace in the apparent darkness of suffering. We enter into a closer relationship and are open to the unpredictability of love, mercy, and grace as we dwell in the darkest times of our lives. We overcome the discomfort of that expectation with fluidity and openness instead of stiffness. "The wind blows where it wills; you hear the sound of it, but you do not know where it comes from or where it is going" (John 3:8).

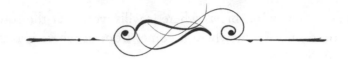

Grace Dispels Darkness

In our world, the probability of our encountering suffering is 100 percent. It is also comforting that God gives us 100 percent of His grace to face it.

Witnessing suffering is unavoidable. We encounter it either directly or indirectly, but it is an unavoidable part of our existence. We see our friends or family members suffering or hear about children dying, wars, hunger, fire, and flooding. Our hearts go out to those who suffer, and we do share in their pain. The road we travel is paved with pitfalls, wants, lacks, distractions, temptations, sickness, and so much more. Everything we do in this world could be in preparation for that ultimate destiny for which we were made.

The ultimate goal is to unite our suffering with God's will in perfect unity to behold His glory. There is no shortcut in life to achieve our purpose of connecting to glory without sacrifice and suffering. As we face the reality of suffering, God made us strong and poured His graces on us so we could withstand temptation. We are on a journey to our ultimate destination, which is the highest glory that is to be revealed after our journey on Earth.

Suffering is disheartening, discouraging, and it can make us lose hope. It can either dim our faith or awaken it. Faith helps us see that no matter the hardship, there is a need to hold on to hope. We see that far and above the agony of winter, spring is on the way with new blooms. This is the grace that sustains us to wait in hope that, in the end, God will bring us into glory. To have this faith in difficult times, we must be open to receive the illuminating light of the Holy Spirit that flows from God's grace unto us. It is in that light that we are able to say, "Father, may Your will be done." God wants us to open our eyes to see this abundance of grace. He does not force us to do it. How do we find untapped grace in our suffering?

What is God telling us through our pain and suffering? It does not always make sense that people should ever undergo the level of hardships many people experience in life. In every instance, there is a mystery being revealed. There is power in God's Word. The profundity of grace dwells in his words. We must explore and discover the abundance of this grace in His Word for us to enjoy the fullness of grace. When we discover the richness of God's goodness that is in His Word and claim it with faith, it dispels the darkness of suffering. Grace draws us closer to tap into the rich goodness that is inherent in God's Word. Suffering has no power over us when the Word of God is alive in us. That is where healing happens, and we grow in our faith.

As love is revealed to us, we wait patiently without complaining. The mystery in suffering is being revealed in the longing of our hearts. The fear and anxiety we go through in times of uncertainty is part of that grace. The encounter with this revealing beauty in suffering is the epiphany that dwells in every tear and cry of anguish we experience.

> I consider that our present sufferings are not worth comparing with the glory that will be revealed in us. For creation waits in eager expectation for the children of God to be revealed. For creation was subjected to frustration, not by its own choice, but by the will of the one who subjected it, in hope that the creation itself will be liberated from its bondage to decay and brought into the freedom and glory of the children of God. (Romans 8:18–21)

Opening our hearts to God's grace dispels the pain we carry in our hearts when we are in the dark. Grace may not end our suffering, but it helps us see things in the new light of glory. This new light gives us new meaning and a foundation for strength and resilience to live on and not despair.

A friend invited me to join their family for dinner at a restaurant. As the time drew closer, I got dressed and was ready to go. I sat on the recliner checking the clock to see when to leave. Time just seemed to fly by. Dinner was great. The first course was a delicious, colorful salad. There was calamari and lobster tail paired with a delicious white wine. The main course was steaming mashed potatoes with a delicious gravy and scrumptious barbeque ribs. Everything looked incredibly delicious. Suddenly my hospital phone rang for an emergency, and it abruptly woke me up from my *dream*! I had actually fallen asleep on the chair while waiting for the right time to leave and had missed dinner. I answered the hospital phone, and it was an emergency for Last Rites. A patient was dying, and the family had requested a priest immediately for Last Rites. I phoned my friends and apologized for missing the dinner. I let them know I was on my way to the hospital for an emergency and would not be able to join them. I didn't have time to fill them in on the details. That was left for another time. I left for the hospital immediately.

When I walked into the room, I was in shock looking at a young lady in her twenties surrounded by different kinds of gigantic machines. Standing by the corner of her feet were the ECMO and ventilator machines mumbling and vibrating. The hemodialysis machine was slowly and quietly humming by the bedside. At the edge of her head stood uncountable IVs of different colors and sizes on a stand like palm tree with their lines gushing out and lying purposelessly on the corner of her pillow. Yet intricately, they were all plugged into every part of her body. I stood there speechless. She was so young with all her endearing dreams and future as a nurse plugged to those machines for survival. I had visited her a couple of times and was hoping and praying for recovery. Now all hope seemed lost since they were about to extubate her. As we prayed the "Hail Mary" that evening, the words "Pray for us sinners now and at the hour of our death" became unbelievably real and alive. With this family, I saw that in their pain, grief, and sorrow, there was an unfathomable grace therein.

Praying for the intercession of the Blessed Virgin Mary at the hour of her death became real and profound. There was an unspoken peace flowing in the hearts of everyone in that room as they said this prayer. There was communion in prayer, and we entered the realm of timelessness by uniting our prayers with those of billions of people around the world. We were praying for our Blessed Mother's intercession to envelope their daughter and the family in her mantle of grace. I gave the young woman the apostolic pardon as required in the rites while still plugged to the machines; then she took one last breath and died.

While absorbed in this sacred moment, the family cried and prayed, held her hands, kissed her lips, and covered her in love. The mother lay on the bed with her, cuddled her, and poured out a river of blessings with her tears while the father softly attempted to overcome his own sorrow to comfort her. The entire family shared the unimaginable bond of grief and loss. They, however, felt God's presence through their prayers. They came to a level of acceptance only possible when our hearts are open to grace. The mother stood up and said, "Death will not have the final word. God will see us through."

These words were grace in its purest form emanating from the darkest moment of their lives. The words were an incarnation of the knowledge that Christ's story does not end on Good Friday. Easter is still on the way. The secret to this family's strength in such a time of anguish was their prayer life. They felt God's presence because they were no strangers to experiencing His mercy and love. The father explained that as a family, they had come to believe in the goodness of God. God had blessed them, and in their loss, God was there with them. He said, "Father, I am living testimony of God's healing miracle and grace. That I am still alive today is through God's mercy. Also, my children were God's answered prayers because we were told that my wife could not conceive. There are mysteries in life that are unexplainable. We felt God's presence even in this darkest hour of our lives. God is ever so present, and it is comforting to know He is here with my family."

I did miss my highly anticipated dinner, but God had prepared a different type of banquet for me. He wanted me to see the power of love, faith, and prayer. He wanted me to see not in an academic sense but in people's faces what Saint Paul meant when he said that love is the greatest gift of all.

God invites us to call upon him in every moment of our lives. He wants to be in relationship with us not only when we are weak or in difficulty. He wants us every day of our lives. He wants us to experience the abundance of His grace both in ourselves and in others as we minister. God never promised us an easy life. There is no separate world for us to live as His children other than the world as we know it. He promised to be with us and share His graces with us in those times when we face difficult situations. What we are invited to do as God's children is tap into God's goodness and grace. He wants to hold us in His glory and wrap us in the palm of His hands in times of danger. We may not always like the outcome. However, when we trust Him, He will take care of us during stormy times.

The apostle Paul exemplified what it means to carry the cross with grace and trust in God. There were times he was afraid. He struggled, he faced trials and persecution, he had a thorn in his flesh and experienced shipwrecks. He was able to withstand all those trials because of his faith and connectedness to God through prayer. We need to understand that as children of God, the things we want may not always flow to us like milk and honey. The truth is that while we live in this world, we will face difficulties and injustice like every other human being. We may feel that what we are going through is too much. Jesus asks us to know that He is there with us and that we should not be afraid. "I have told you these things, so that in me you may have peace. In this world you will have trouble. But take heart! I have overcome the world" (John 16:33).

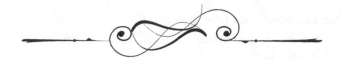

The Ministry of Compassion

We know the effect medicine has on our bodies while we strive to heal and recover. What is the role of prayer when the doctors and nurses are taking charge of our health? Why pray to God when I have my medicine? In all honesty, between the doctors and the scientific breakthroughs, we do have better life expectancies. Even with so many diseases and illnesses in the world, people still live longer and better lives despite their health conditions. We have machines that can work as well as our own hearts to keep people alive. There are better medicines these days to manage our health, liver, kidneys, and any other part of the body that were unavailable in the not-so-distant past. These advancements extend our lives more than anyone could have ever imagined thirty years ago. Medicine can control brain function, muscles, pain, and even our emotions. It can bring supreme comfort to those dying. Through modern medicine, transplanting major organs is becoming commonplace. We see why it would feel like a waste of time to pray to God when we are at the hospital. Why do we want God to do for us what medicine could do for us?

Understanding the world like this would lead to fierce contention between science and faith. In this case, science would be more reliable and productive than faith. A battle of supremacy between scientific and technological growth and faith in the Supreme Being is currently raging. A die is cast between science in its empirical, verifiable achievements and the absurdity of a delusional faith in a God who is omnipotent and omnipresent and perpetually absent to human perception. This becomes the scientific opposition to faith and the sense of mystery because humans have the potential to achieve this greatness without God. Hence, we see that doctors and medicines are reliable and dependable while God is not. Why do we need to waste our time praying to God instead of doing what we can and trusting doctors to fix us? If doctors were unable to help, we would know our luck had run out, and there would be nothing further to do.

The Hospital, a Home of Compassion

Compassion is clearly the foundation of the hospital healing ministry. It is a place where care providers are called to show compassion to those who are sick and weak. We all share in this unique characteristic to show compassion to those suffering whether as scientists or by supporting patients through prayers. Compassion is the primary motivating factor for the ministry at the hospital. *Compassion* originates from Latin: *com-*, "together," and *pati*, "suffer"—*suffer with*. We suffer with patients as they suffer by being present and reaching out to them. While the doctors and nurses show compassion by providing medicine to ease a patient's pain, I choose to suffer with those who are suffering by offering comfort and consolation to them. I share their sacred space with them. I listen to people in pain, their fear, loneliness, anxiety, abandonment, and frustrations because these experiences have a direct impact on their ability to respond to the treatment they receive at the hospital.

Doing my clinical hours as a CPE resident at the hospital, I witnessed a deep faith, dedication, love, and compassion in many doctors. This experience dismantled the myth I had grown up believing that doctors are detached and practical while dealing with patients. I thought they were trained not to express feelings of sympathy. I thought it was believed that such emotion would interfere with the objectivity of their work. The same can be assumed about the work of a chaplain or a priest at the hospital by believing that their "job" is to provide Last Rites and send people to heaven. I laugh when I encounter so many people who ask me, "What do you really do at the hospital? What is your job with patients apart from doing Last Rites?" Many doctors are surprised when I tell them that, as chaplains, we make "spiritual assessments" to provide quality care to patients.

Working at the hospital gave me the opportunity to see love in the heart of the doctors. While doing palliative rounds with some doctors, I saw another side that was compassionate and vulnerable. I have seen doctors cry, especially in cases involving children. I have enjoyed jokes, laughter, and humor with them. It was eye-opening to see the human quality we all share. I also witnessed the healing gift nurses offer to patients on a daily basis as their bedside angels. I was part of the healing mercy shared by every chaplain, psychologist, social worker, music and harp therapist, patient advocate, and other staff at the hospital. The hospital is a place we need to share in this expression of compassion.

When I walk through the halls of the hospital to pray for people, I am not in competition with medicine and all the marvelous work that medical teams do. Faith enriches medicine to provide a caring service that is meaningful to patients and their families. Everyone at the hospital is, in one way or another, involved in the healing ministry and supports the patient's recovery and well-being. It is in that spirit of caring that we, as the faith community, join the medical team in providing support and pastoral care to enrich the patient's experience. Initially, we are present with the patient to offer comfort, love, and prayers as they go through the distress of being at the hospital. The medical professionals may not have the training, time, and patience to provide this pastoral service that will offer the meaningful support patients need in the most critical time of distress.

I was once called up at midnight to visit a patient for Last Rites. When I was told his name and room, I knew he was the same patient who was anointed during the day. As a feeling being, I was reluctant to go back; but focused on the anguish his family was undoubtedly experiencing, I went. When I got there, I spoke with the patient's nurse to get a clear picture of the prognosis. The nurse clearly stated, "We maximized every medication for him as his blood pressure keeps dropping."

With this knowledge, I went in to pray for him. I asked the family what they wanted me to do. The daughter answered that I should pray for him and give him Last Rites because they were not sure what would happen if he had to go in for another surgery. I said the prayers and invited the family to share a moment in prayer with the patient. From the information I got from the nurse, I knew they were finding it difficult to process the situation. "I invite you to share a moment of personal time and prayer with him. I want you to treasure the moment you are sharing with him. Your hope and prayers are not in vain because the love you are sharing with him is something that you will never regret. I know that you love him and want what is best for him. But you still have to ask yourself what, if any, would his quality of life be should he undergo yet another surgery. The doctors are best suited to provide information about that. At some point, one has to give oneself permission to let our loved one go precisely because we love them."

Accompanying the family to share quality time during that sacred moment was important. It was a good feeling to journey with them during the transition from "I did not fight hard enough to keep my husband alive" to "In my hurt, I chose to honor him by allowing him to go with dignity." When the attending doctor came back to check with the family about the care plan, the conversation went smoothly. The family agreed not to pursue any aggressive treatments if they would not help him get better. He died peacefully within a few hours.

I strongly believe that the medical team would have found it difficult to guide this family through their decision as they would have felt they were letting their loved one down. Ministering to them brought comfort and a clearer perspective to this family when faced with the reality of their father's impending death. The doctors and the medical staff were doing everything possible to show compassion to this patient and offer support to this family. They did everything humanly possible for this patient, even working with the chaplaincy team to provide comfort to the patient and his family. Through faith, this patient was honored, and the family was able to let him go. The entire experience was meaningful to them.

Faith Advances and Enriches Medicine

From the origin of science to the modern age, many great scientists were Christians. People like Nicolaus Copernicus, Galileo Galilei, Isaac Newton, and an endless list of generations of successful scientists who were devoted Christians used their knowledge in science to build a better world. Science and faith should work together. Grace perfects nature, as Saint Thomas Aquinas would say. Everything we use in the scientific world, our knowledge, and the scientific discoveries we have are graces given to us by God. They are gifts we received from grace to build a better world for ourselves and others. All the medicines we use at the hospital are all gifts of nature. With the use of our human intelligence, we are able to utilize these gifts of nature to enhance the human condition. We are converting herbs into chemical components that enhance the human condition.

One morning during breakfast, I was sharing my experiences at the hospital with another priest. I had a patient the previous day who said he did not need any prayers. He believed that God has nothing to do with his getting better. He said the doctors have all the knowledge for him to be well and God has no part in it. As Friedrich Nietzsche said, "God is dead. We killed Him." So we should be doing things for ourselves without Him as He is no longer needed in this twenty-first century. The priest told me the story of a contest between God and the scientists.

Scientists, laughing, called God and told Him, "Sorry, God, we don't need You anymore. We are now able to take care of our health very well. We have machines and medications that can do anything we want in our human body. We can treat any wound and restore health in people. We have developed laser machines that could do surgeries with zero margin of error. We have artificial intelligence, which is unaided learning and corrects its own mistakes to improve itself. We do brain surgeries to restore people to health for things we used to think were impossible. We can clone anyone we want and modify people to get the exact personality we want without Your intervention. When we want to travel, we have supersonic jets that can take us comfortably to any part of the world. We go to Mars and to some other planets. Everything people used to pray to You before, we can now do for ourselves. Thanks for Your help, but we are good without You."

God asked the scientists, "Let's have a contest. If you win, I retire. You can then do whatever you want. Let us create any human, body parts, an arm, leg, eye, or head, anything you want."

The scientists said, "That is easy. We have the machines that could modify clay and get the exact synthetic texture we want to get the muscle as we want it. We are always improving on the previous experiences, and we will surely get there."

The scientists began the competition. They brought the materials, the clay, the chemicals, the tools and started testing the tools and what would work and not work. They activated the electrical current and modified the textures to make it feel like a human body and began to work.

God called out to them and said, "Stop, my friend. Everything you are using belongs to Me. They were all created by Me. The clay, the rock you want to modify to give you the bone texture, the chemicals you want to use were from the herbs that I created. I made mine out of nothing. You should start yours out of nothing. I created out of nothing, and I expect you as experts to start yours out of nothing too. That would be the only way you could be my match." The end!

A patient told me, "Thanks for your prayers. Receiving communion today was what I needed. I am happy also for the advancement in health science. Without it, there is no way I would be alive today." Pointing to his Left Ventricular Assist Device (LVAD) that he carried around to help improve blood flow from the heart through the body, he said, "I have carried this LVAD for more than nine years. I would be dead without it. God is with me and has seen me through it all. It was showing a yellow light, and I called. I was asked to come over and have it checked. I am happy for the grace God gave me. He used these doctors to sustain me. I am grateful."

It was incredible to hear his testimony, which blended his faith in God with the quality medical care he was receiving. It made me proud of the doctors and every staff member working at the hospital. It gave me profound joy to confirm the need for spiritual support that is at times neglected at the hospital. It is very important that we understand that science and faith are not in opposition. They are given to us as graces to enhance our living conditions on earth. Science and faith have to work together to build a better world. This gift of knowledge and nature is a manifestation of God's grace to humanity. All research, enhanced treatment, expedient surgery that allows for a higher level of success is a gift of grace. We received these gifts to build a better world, and it does not imply that we are mightier than the giver. As the saying goes, "doctors treat, God cures." We take the medication; it is God who helps those medications work in our human form. We must know that clarity and objectivity in science do not always work when it comes to finding a meaning behind our conditions and situations.

Hospital ministry requires teamwork. One day, I was tending to a Catholic patient, and a resident doctor walked into the room and started talking to the patient. She marched into the room in the middle of our conversation without even acknowledging that someone was already there with the patient. I was upset and almost walked away had it not been for the patient. The patient was informed that the fluid being drained from her feet was cancerous. It had already infected her bones and bloodstream. She was told she had a few months to live. She was narrating these experiences when the doctor walked in and started asking her about her medications and checking her vital signs.

The patient apologized when she left. The conversation I had with her went on for more than one hour. The grace of God allowed me to be a companion for this woman in this moment of brokenness. She cried, and I allowed her to pour out her brokenness and grief. When I finished my visit with her, she said, "Thanks, Father, for what you did for me. This is the greatest thing that has happened since I heard the news." I thanked her and left. Every doctor should understand that their work is special in the healing ministry. However, there are so many other little angels who are also part of this team. Grace implies that we need one another to work together in the fight against sicknesses. No department could do it alone. No one should feel they have the monopoly on healing. We need one another, and this cannot be overemphasized. The doctors are important, the nurses, the cleaners, those keeping the records, the chaplains, social workers, and all other offices offering support.

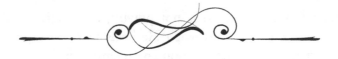

The Efficiency of Prayer

Everyone we meet, irrespective of what image they portray, struggles. They may not always come to us to announce it, but we all have our share of suffering. We have crosses to bear, be in sickness, disease, pandemic, mental illness, drug addiction, alcohol, no job, poverty—the list is endless. Everywhere we go, every office we enter, and every job we do, we can see people struggling in different ways. "Be alert and of sober mind. Your enemy the devil prowls around like a roaring lion looking for someone to devour" (1 Peter 5:8). What is our response in times of temptation and persecution? Do we fight to defend ourselves? Are we not required to turn the other cheek as Jesus Christ taught us? How do we reconcile, accepting our sickness as the will of God and praying for God's healing power? Many saints handed over their suffering to God in atonement for the suffering of others and the sins of the world. Are we not supposed to see our suffering as the will of God and accept it as the saints did? Should we pray for healing as Jesus did when He asked God His Father "remove this cross from me!"? Like Jesus while doing all within our power also asking God for healing is likewise necessary. We should not passively accept sickness as the will of God.

When I visit with patients, I do pray for the doctors, nurses, and staff working to help patients at the hospital. I pray for God to help these doctors, nurses, and every care provider in the performance of their duties. I do pray that all complications, confusions, and mistakes be avoided by the medical team as they look after these patients. I pray for God to use the medicines, food, and liquid administered to patients as a means of healing to help them with their recovery. I always pray that while patients are at the hospital, everyone setting foot in their rooms would be an angel of healing to support them.

Praying at the hospital is not praying for magic. God is not a magician. There are times when He heals in an unexpected way. When that happens, it goes beyond any scientific method, so we call that a miracle. God has performed so many miracles through prayers of healing. God's Word is real and powerful. He gives life to His people in their times of need. God bestows the grace of healing for the glory of His name. Unfortunately, the sacrament of the anointing of the sick may easily be performed without faith or expectation of any possible healing from God. The sacrament not only provides comfort and consolation, but it is actually a prayer to God for real healing of the sick and not something done as the fulfilment of a ritual. There have been so many instances when God has had a direct hand in the healing process and expedited the recovery of the sick. All hands are on deck to fight sickness and offer succor to the sick.

I recently received a thank-you card that I want to share:

> Dear Father, about three weeks ago, I was a patient at Hershey Med. for a brain biopsy. You came to see me and spoke so lovely to me, and I just wanted to thank you so much for your visit. You gave me Holy Communion, and I haven't had it for thirty years. As it turns out, I have a fatal tumor in my brain, and I will be coming back to the hospital for six weeks of radiation and chemo. I am asking for you to pray for me if you would. I will need all of God's mercy to deal with this. Again, thank you, Father. You were my guardian angel that day. God bless you in your work. Sincerely.

What other attestation do we need to show the importance of faith in the healing ministry at the hospital? The condition of this patient, as she stated it, was terminal. However, she felt compelled to share her testimony of the comfort she received while being cared for. It is not always easy for us Catholics to share testimonies of God's goodness due to fear of being considered prideful. It is important, however, to allow the grace of God to manifest itself because it is never about us. God is reaching out to His people and giving them His graces. The instrument He is using to do that is still unworthy and flawed. I, as His instrument, am in need of His grace because of that.

After Mass one Sunday, as I was greeting some of the people who had attended, I saw a woman hanging around. When there were fewer people left, she walked up to me. "Father, I know you do not remember me. I was at the hospital in Hershey last month. You came to anoint me. I don't know how it happened, but you brought so much comfort and peace to me. I was really stressed out and was scared. As I wept, you stayed by me even in my pain. Your prayer was so profound that I just cried when you left. I felt God's presence throughout the night. I was so surprised the next day, I was healed. I felt the Word of God alive in me, and I felt God's healing touch that night. I was discharged the next day. I just want to say, thanks so much. You are special."

On another occasion, I was called to give the Last Rites to a mother. It broke my heart when I saw how young the mother looked. It was so painful to imagine what all her children were going through at that moment as one of them was a pediatrician and the other a nurse. They could not offer any help to prevent their mother from dying. It would be far easier to perform the Last Rites and remind them that God is taking their mother to heaven. However, I felt their pain, and I allowed my heart to express the depth of my love and appreciation for what they offered their mother in their brokenness. "You are hurting right now because you love your mother with all your heart. It hurts so much to see her in this condition and knowing that there is nothing you can do to help. I wish to remind you that even then, you are choosing to stand by her. You choose to honor her. You choose to give her dignity and respect. She may not be able to say a word to you, but remember, your presence means a lot to her. You are blessing her with your presence and tears. Those tears are your expression of love and do not mean that you are feeble. I wish to invite you to take your time and pray for her from your heart. Say those prayers and mean them. Allow her to bless you too as you do that."

After all that, I went home. The next day, I happened to be visiting a patient near their room, and I decided to check on them. They were so glad that I had stopped by. One of the sisters said, "Father, thanks so much for your gift yesterday. I know my mother is dying. Your words gave me peace yesterday. For the first time in weeks, I slept for nine hours, and my sister said she slept for more than seven hours. That has not happened in ages. We are ready now. You brought so much peace to my mother. When you finished, all the wrinkles on her face and expressions of stress relaxed immediately. We are so glad that you were such a blessing to my family last night."

As we are all involved in fighting sickness and disease, we are also open to learn, grow, and welcome innovation. Grace means we are not a finished product. I am so happy that I can be part of this grace-sharing mission of healing. We all give support to those who are sick and to their families as they search for meaning and grace themselves in times of suffering. Even though we are an integral part of this ministry of grace, we are still in need of grace. The doctors, nurses, as well as the entire staff at the hospital, need grace to function because we share in our vulnerability. The patients who are suffering will do well to pray for anyone who sets foot in their rooms. A little prayer asking for blessings for them would go a long way to heal their spirit. Millions of anonymous workers do their jobs to make healing possible. They may never come face-to-face with patients and are never told thank-you. Please know that God sees their passion to serve, love, and care for others. By doing what they do, they are part of the army of healing angels at the hospital who fight against every sickness and disease to bring healing graces to others. I hope they pay attention, and when they get home tired and worn-out, they can hear God saying, *Thank you.*

I feel the ministry at the hospital and many other services we provide for one another is being Christlike. Doctors, nurses, and other staff want their patients to get well. Many times, we say a quiet prayer in our hearts. Those are profound prayers even though we do not fall to our knees. We show mercy, love, and compassion without realizing it. There are many of angels who are working around the clock in the healing ministry to ensure our recovery. Walking into patients' rooms has opened my eyes to the grace of God manifested through all the staff at the hospital. The nurses are archangels who minister to patients, giving them their medication and caring for them. These angels do not always realize that they are a source of God's abundant grace to those who they encounter. God opens my eyes to His graces through the various departments at the hospital. There are many hidden angels taking care of the logistics of the administration, paperwork, cleaning, financing, supervising, and making sure that everything works well for the patient's well-being. Therefore, my use of the word *grace* carries a wider scope. At the hospital, grace is in everything and everywhere. Everything is grace.

The Phenomenon of Rediscovery

As a chaplain working in the hospital, everyone expects me to believe and have faith in God because I represent God. What God do I represent if I do not find God myself? Is it a God who is transcendent and separate from human existence? Is it an omnipotent, abstract God who is in heaven and has nothing to do with this imperfect world? How do I offer hope to those carrying their cross on their hospital bed if I do not experience grace myself? How do I give a meaningful answer to those suffering if I cannot find a meaningful answer myself? Hope is only possible in my ability to find and encounter God, who is there with us all in the hospital and in humanity. It is God who shares the cross with me, wipes away my tears, and tells me it is okay to cry. It is God who makes me realize that questioning while hurting does not mean I do not believe. God lets me know that my faith is searching for meaning and seeking understanding. When I feel I am in the dark, I theologize and reach out to God because my faith seeks understanding.

While reflecting on finding meaning and answers to our pain, how do we know that God cares? Instead of accepting the deflected theological answers that are readily available to escape the reality of the pain and anguish I see daily, I search for the God who is alive and present. A God who is not only on the cross but who is with the patient "nailed" to their sick bed. I find a God who walks along with me as I watch patients in their brokenness and vulnerability. I want a God who cares to cry with us throughout the night when we are hurting. I prefer a God who is not ashamed of us when we wet our pillows with tears of agony. *Akwa ariri*. We want Jesus to answer our prayers and heal all those who are sick as we cry out to Him. I love the Jesus who loves us as friends. I love the one who is not ashamed to share in our humanity and helps us through His grace. I love the fact that Jesus cries, feels our pain, and is always there to save, heal, protect, and provide for us.

This experience was humbling because I allowed myself to walk into a patient's sacred space. This was the grace that broke me. I became present with those who suffer. I shared in the suffering with others. When I opened my heart to this grace and the mystery therein, I didn't realize God had a different plan. He drew me closer to Himself by piercing my heart, and it made me hunger for Him more and more. He made me see the beauty in the body of those who are sick even in their vulnerability and brokenness. The deeper agony of pain and anguish patients were experiencing was transformed into grace because God was present to change the unpleasant smells into a beautiful fragrance. These experiences with patients at the hospital humbled me, to say the least. I learned to walk in fear and trembling. We were always told to carry our crosses. When the weight of the cross is too heavy to bear, we should learn to cry out to God for help and support. This cry is part of prayer and grace.

Those questions that frightened me at the beginning of my ministry as chaplain at the hospital were legitimate. In my reflections, I also found some answers to which God was calling my attention: do you want to allow death to have the upper hand or final say in your life? Don't give the key of your life to sickness, sadness, and disease to determine what gives you joy. You have to open your eyes to see that the resurrection is not about a future experience of resurrection of the dead. It is the resurrection that is happening here and now. It is your resurrection in brokenness. It is your experience of the abundance of grace. It is your ability to rise and find bliss for yourself even in the deepest darkness. It is the ability to rise again from the ashes and conquer death with love and mercy.

The power of grace in each and every one of us is resurrection here on earth. Everyone at the hospital has to know that regardless of what they may be going through, we have the powerful witnesses of sisters and brothers around the world. They are praying and interceding for us. It is the resurrection that shows that we are alive in the hearts of hundreds of people who have been touched by our smiles, love, and even tears. It is the hundreds of people we invite into our sacred space to experience the mystery of our brokenness. It is the resurrection in timelessness that is grace in abundance. This is the power of the resurrection that even death cannot steal from us. That is why Saint Paul states, "What is it that will separate us from the love of God. Is it sickness, suffering, pain and death? No!" (Romans 8:23–38). See that I weep with you, and I am in every one of those tears falling from your eyes. Millions of angels are in tears because of you. You are never alone. I am with you. See me through your tears.

As I witnessed the suffering and pain people face daily at the hospital, I was in awe at the abundance of inner grace that each one of them has in those trying times. This experience with suffering opened my heart to the amazing beauty being revealed in the lives of every patient I meet at the hospital as they carry their daily crosses. The revealed beauty is the total surrender of our humanity to one another as we experience grace. At the hospital bed, it is hard to know who is a lawyer, a senator, a teacher, a bishop, a janitor, or a mechanic. We all share the common denominator that holds us together—being human and having flesh and blood. This grace dwelling in every patient broke the walls of expectations in me. It opened my eyes to see that there is more than meets the eye in every person going through suffering. Having to face the pain of children and young people dying frightened me. There was nothing I could do to bring them back to their parents, who were in tears.

The Marvelous Gift of Tears

I search for my own answers as I face suffering on a daily basis. I want to understand its meaning and relevance in life. I want to know that, as a child of God, I am important to God. I want to know that I matter, that my life matters, that my opinion matters, and that my being matters to God. It is necessary to realize that when we process the situation, search for answers and meaning, finding these answers for ourselves provides more healing than what any person could ever tell us. Suffering is not always as clear as we are made to believe, and neither is the solution as easy to come by. That is why these questions are authentic to me. Some of my expressions may appear disparaging, but that is how I feel when I see those tears while standing by the hospital beds. These questions mean a lot to those I see every day—those who are broken like me, facing the reality of our humanness and suffering.

How do we behold this beauty in emptiness and brokenness amidst immense suffering? Where can we find grace when crushed by pain? Where is the strength to keep going on as we face brokenness, betrayal, and humiliation? As a priest, being at the hospital and witnessing pain and suffering gave me the grace of being broken and experiencing my own vulnerability. Being at the hospital offered me another grace. It was the grace to give myself permission to cry, to laugh, to be broken, and to question God. I was able to express my deepest pain and anguish without feeling that I was not "supposed" to.

We were told that God is right there with us during storms and darkness. We feel the joy of speaking to God in times of suffering when we exclaim, "Please, God, let me see You! Let me feel You! Show me something that would let me know that You are with me, O God! Don't remain silent while we are crushed and shaken!" The grace to enjoy the gift of peace, not holding on to fear and worry about right or wrong, is the grace to see Jesus by our side at the darkest hours. It is the grace to embrace a new language of expressing that which is genuine and authentic. A flowing river so liberating and refreshing from which we are purposefully kept away—it is the language of *tears*.

Witnessing daily suffering at the hospital broke the shield of my ministering with priestly authority as I did with the sacraments. Suffering opened the door for grace so the sacraments became a joint celebration for the patient and priest. I surrendered myself in humility. I accepted my humanity and that I am as imperfect and vulnerable as every patient. We truly share in the sacrament of healing together as we are all in need of God's healing. My priestly authority was blessed by grace while present where there is daily suffering and pain. Being in the presence of suffering allowed the sacrament to be a moment when both priest and patient alike asked for the grace of God to allow healing for all. Much like when Jesus came to this earth and shared in our humanity and suffered, I could see the same in patients. We all suffer, are sick, and in need of healing. Everyone at the hospital shares in this. We are in the midst of it together. We all experience turmoil while searching for God's mercy, who is the ultimate healer. It was humbling to accept that I was struggling to find meaning behind all that suffering.

Like a child afraid of stepping into water, I opened my heart to grace to step into my river of fear. When I started working at the hospital, I was afraid of not saying the right thing or doing the right thing. However, my experiences at the hospital were opening me up to the abundance of grace. It expunged the fear of shame, the anguish, and the struggle to say the right thing in the midst of suffering. It was a staggering revelation for me to realize the sheer inadequacy of the answers I thought I had to explain suffering, pain, and the crosses people carry. Now I feel I can be me without feeling ashamed or having to do what is expected when I am broken. As I witness people suffering and in pain, I give myself permission to pour my heart out to God without feeling badly. I am becoming freer daily as I express my fears and brokenness to God as I am. I am able to immerse myself in this new language of love in the uncontrollable tears that flow from my heart in those times of anguish.

This grace is so freeing that my heart overflows with joy and love even in my vulnerability. I accepted my brokenness and no longer worried about the misconception that crying with those who suffer was "not priestly." I enjoyed the grace and the beauty of having had my eyes opened by God. I now enjoy God's special grace and am not worried about saying or doing what is expected when the gift of tears is manifested. It is so liberating to enjoy this power of the Holy Spirit and tap into these graces. The gift of tears is the greatest language of love.

When Jesus heard of the death of His friend Lazarus, He wept. He grieved for him. His heart went out to him to express the pain He was going through at that moment. Saint John, in this narrative, offered a lengthy discourse to show how this particular short verse and act was the center of Jesus's manifestation of His love. Yet he presents us with the discourse of the Jews who were observing Him and analyzing His actions: "See how He loved him!" But some of them said, "Could not He who opened the eyes of the blind man have kept this man from dying?" (John 11:35–37). Jesus was deeply moved with compassion and love. He was there with Lazarus and the family through it all even when they were not aware of God's presence. He shared in the brokenness with them even with the knowledge of the type of miracle He intended to perform. "Did I not tell you that if you believe, you will see the glory of God?" (John 11:40).

In times of suffering, I accept that my limitations are not something to be ashamed of but a means to glorify God. My weakness, my brokenness, my vulnerability, and my questioning no longer cause me embarrassment; I see them as grace. It is through the eyes of grace that I allow myself to share my struggles and vulnerability doing my ministry at the hospital. I am not here to join theodicy conversations and defend God. I do not share in these questions because I am losing my faith. I am presenting them for us to know that we are all in this struggle together. I am offering myself up just as I am without being ashamed of doing so. My faith is seeking understanding so I can be an authentic witness to God's love for people in the most vulnerable moments of their lives.

When I place the burden of those I love and care about in God's hands through prayer, I do it knowing that God is with me in that space of darkness, vulnerability, and grace. I found grace in not running away in the face of suffering and pain. I cry out to God these days and share with Him how I feel about His silence. It is freeing, and I feel refreshed after pouring my heart out to Him. I do not feel ashamed or afraid that I should not be saying this or that to God. I just cry out to Him and say exactly what I feel. That is what matters most. I enjoy the sacred relationship with God in my brokenness. So He allows me to experience grace and beauty in that silent darkness which surrounds me. Grace does not remove the reality of our internal struggles.

The Pinnacle of the Revelation

The grace God bestows upon me on a daily basis enables me to share in people's pain and brokenness. I see that Jesus is with those who suffer, and He is suffering with them. I step into patients' rooms with reverence for them and in admiration for their strength. It makes me pay attention, be a better listener and understand that suffering is senseless but does not have to be meaningless. Is it possible that God just wants us to be in relationship with Him during that silence and brokenness? Could it be that He is not really interested in providing us with an explanation of why He is doing whatever He does? Could we be okay with not worrying about making sense of all our plights? While at the hospital, is God trying to speak to us in different ways? Is He ministering to us through the doctors, nurses, and medicine? When we look out the window, are we paying attention to God's presence? Do we keep repeating what we think we know about suffering like a beautiful caged parrot?

Being at the hospital, I find I am not the wise counselor who is there to offer guidance and direction to patients. These experiences have broken my bones, my heart, and my strength. I have come to accept patients who, in that space, are not able to act as they are expected. I enter that space as they invite me, praying and hoping for healing for them. I am no longer God's ambassador bringing God to them for healing. I am with them in their pain and affliction, and my heart breaks with theirs. Together we cry. Together we raise our eyes up to God in prayer. Together we hurt, and together we search for answers. Grace allows me to be at the hospital, praying and asking Jesus to heal us all.

When we are at the hospital and we sincerely pray from our hearts and not just with our lips, it provides much comfort to patients. As a result, God has continuously answered our prayers. God's answers to our prayers may not always be as we expect. We pray and expect miracles every time. My question was, does God answer and grant us those miracles? I have realized that the answer is *yes*. But what do these miracles look like?

Maybe the miracle is for us to have the courage to say, "God, may Your will be done." It may entail giving honor to our loved ones by allowing them to die peacefully and have peace ourselves as we freely embrace their passing while knowing that we will be okay. Maybe the pinnacle of grace, even in that horror, is to allow them to go with dignity instead of subjecting them to trials and experimental surgeries. It is the moment when we realize that we love them enough to let them go as we accept that their condition is irreversible, and they will have no quality of life. The miracle may be the gift of peace during those last moments. The miracle may be the expression of the indestructible love as we bless them with the abundance of our tears flowing like rivers.

The pinnacle of this revelation may be this sensational feeling of peace that envelops us when we realize that our loved one lived a meaningful life regardless of age and is going in peace to see God and all those who died before us. This does not imply that we feel their impending physical absence any less or that we can actually be happy they will be in heaven instead of here among us. It means that we are in communion with our loved ones and are moving on *with* them as they transition into eternal life. They are part of our being and will remain within and in us. They will always be alive in our memories. It is imperative for us to find our own voices, grace, language, and that which gives meaning to everything in the midst of suffering. We reclaim the light in our spirit when change is afoot instead of settling for self-pity. We fight the urge to submit by default to submission and despair. Sharing this sacred time is boldly enriching and the pin-nacle of a revelation that helps us carry on as we wait to be reunited with them one day. It is the light of this glory that will accompany us for as long as we live.

We are not God's angels of death sending people to heaven. We are God's angels of healing. As we set foot in a patient's room and see them lying on that bed, we are not immune to their despair. It touches our hearts, and we pray. As we now know, healing does not consist of just prayers or just medicine. They are not mutually exclusive. When we pray at the hospital, we pray with and for doctors, the entire staff, and ultimately for the patient's healing. We need to pray from our hearts as we speak to God on behalf of those who are suffering.

Unfortunately, some priests do not believe in the efficacy of the sacrament we are carrying out. We may see it as something that we have to do because it is required. I watched in dismay a priest answering a question about the usefulness of the sacrament of the anointing of the sick. He answered, "It is to make people feel good and feel supported. If they are dying and can't do confession, it forgives their sins." When he was asked if he ever believed God could heal anyone because He gave them this anointing, he answered in the negative, "No!" Unfortunately, he had not transcended the book knowledge to experience God's healing mercy in his ministry. It would make no sense to be woken up at 2:00 a.m. to go to the hospital only for "feel-good session." If the sacrament had no other efficacy, why call a priest?

Many saints were able to open their hearts to the grace of God as they went through suffering. That is the grace I seek and search for. I had not been able to find the meaningful God in theoretical answers provided by speculative theology. I felt it intellectualized suffering and made God an abstract and distant entity detached from our everyday suffering. Such proposition seemed empty and meaningless because it did not bring the patient's story into the conversation. I am not in any way represented in the experience of such a God. I try to find God and have access to the God that is meaningful to me. I am looking for a God who cares for me and is there with me in the dreadful moment when I cannot come up with the right words.

Working at the hospital is a grace for me. Grace is no longer as straightforward and clear as I once thought it to be. Grace could disappear at any given time, yet it is grace. My understanding of God's grace at the hospital is no longer the mere expectation of God answering our prayers the way we want. I find God's unfathomable grace when I feel He did not answer because He is there. It is an exceptional privilege to serve people at the most vulnerable time of their lives. I cannot trade the grace I find these days in my terrifying struggle. In those times of unpredictable anguish and anxiety experienced by patients dwells grace. There is horror in grace as there is grace in horror. They are inseparable.

It is the humility to accept our limitations and weaknesses and still see them as grace that matters. The emptiness in brokenness and the openness that I saw in the heart of patients I came across was remarkable. This brokenness opens the heart of every patient going through pain to find the grace that the angel Gabriel saw in Mary, the mother of Jesus, when he said, "Hail Mary, full of grace." I see the heavens open and the glory of God coming down to fill our hearts with the assurance of God's presence. In those sacred times of prayer, God is ever present.

I realize that in times of suffering, heaven is no longer something that is yet to come. Heaven is here and now while we are still in a dark sacred space. In poetic terms, I start hearing God's voice manifested in the lovely flowers placed by a patient's window saying, *You are not alone! I am with you always and will be until the end of your hospital stay*. The birds flying across the window also serve as reminders of life beyond this earth. The medicine dropping continuously through the IV into a patient's body seems like an agent of grace. These things represent God's grace as He ministers to patients while being restored to wholeness. Lord, You forgive our sins by Your mercy, and you do not judge us because You love us. You are dwelling in the hearts of those covered by hospital sheets, and that is where heaven and earth meet.

Love and faithfulness meet; righteousness and
peace kiss each other. Faithfulness springs forth

from earth, and righteousness looks down from heaven. The Lord will indeed give what is good, and our land will yield its harvest. Righteousness goes before him and prepares the way for his steps. (Psalm 85:10–13)

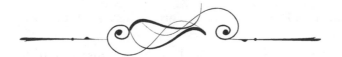

Conclusion

At the hospital, patients are covered by white sheets to hide their wounds. They are in pain, but the pain is either masked or concealed. We are not supposed to see that underneath the white sheet are the bloodstained bandages, the reddened skin, or the worst of their conditions. We are not usually allowed to see the tears. During those times when they struggle with their faith, they are afraid to verbalize those feelings for fear of judgment. Many of the visitors who come in to offer their support expect patients in their sickbed to be and remain positive and optimistic. Expressions of pain, fear, and concern are seldom discussed, if not outright repressed. Visitors avoid delicate subjects or addressing the inevitable. The result is patients finding themselves alone and dejected trying to find answers and clamoring to God for help.

It is easy to spout phrases like, "Believe and have faith," "Don't ask God why," "It must be the will of God," "God took your child to be one of his beautiful angels in heaven," "Everything happens for a reason," "Your suffering is for a purpose," when we really do not have anything better to say. Unfortunately, these are porous patriarchal, theological propositions that fail to address the real issues. It is the theology we are expected to echo and what we have been told. Faith is deemed a finished project, and we just have to accept and absorb it. If this were the case, little would it matter what our own stories have taught us and what God has been teaching us along our journeys and specially at the end of it. It is a theology that fails to remember that we are individuals created in God's image and likeness. It is a theology devoid of love and mercy. My story, my pain, my tears, my fears, and my being are uniquely mine. I am part of a people, a culture, a community, and a generation. My individual existence is vital and holds an important place in the group because I am distinct and a blessing.

Without faith, it is difficult to have a meaningful foundation to deal with suffering. I reflect on the mystery of human suffering through the lens of our Christian faith. I bemoan powerlessness in times of suffering. The language of love is the greatest gift we have to reconnect us both to ourselves and to the person suffering. Words fail to convey this expression of indestructible love. It is important to allow those who suffer to see us broken and hurting. That is more meaningful than any hopeful or encouraging words spoken. Grace dispels our darkest experiences and elevates them to a new level of peace. This grace is shared by all in the ministry of compassion.

We seek to understand just like Thomas did when he said, "Unless I put my fingers on his side, I refuse to believe." This reflection and questioning represent our unwillingness to accept *no* for an answer from God, who is our Father. He made us in His own image and likeness. I am not willing to join the crowd in their belief system. I want to experience faith on a personal level. I want to put my own fingers on Jesus's side to experience Him as He is. Is He real? Is He to be trusted? Does God really care? Does He know we are in pain and that every night our pillows are soaked with tears and our eyes red as we cry for help?

I refuse to be part of that obnoxious spirituality or theological framework that claims to know it all. I am no longer interested in the intellectual, abstract, ineffable God who is all-knowing but uncaring. I do not want a god who keeps all the answers to himself and for whom my reasoning is irrelevant. I am not interested in a god who knows why I suffer and does not care to tell me why. I want the real God, the God who listens to my heart and soul and who is there with me in my suffering. I prefer the God who is patient with me in my foolishness and cares for me as I am. I want Him who loves me in that messy place and helps me get out of there. I am afraid of a god where only a few partake in the monopoly of knowing him while the rest of us wobble and fumble around in ignorance. I want the God who cares to journey with me in the deepest abyss and leads me out of it. He is not the god who is angry with me because I am not perfect. He is the God who created me to be *me* and wants me to be me as I serve Him. In being me, He draws me closer to Himself. That is the God I find in Jesus Christ, who left the glory of heaven to share in our humanness, sickness, and suffering. He accepted to be born in a stable surrounded by animals and manure. He cares for me and is not ashamed to call me His brother. He rejoiced with His disciples and friends and also cried with them when they suffered. He is the God I want to worship and adore because He shares in the tears of every patient lying on a hospital bed.

I find meaning and relevance in connecting with God as I am, not as others want. I know that God feels that the voice He gave me is good enough. He allows me to use that voice as it is because my own voice is important to him. In times of sickness, we all come together irrespective of our ages, titles, and ranks. We come to be with the one who experienced brokenness on our behalf: Jesus Christ. That is the God who dares to dwell in us with our broken spirits and broken bodies. He is the God that took a risk to be with the rejected, the outcasts, women, children, the sick, and the sinners. He is not the god that only dwells in imposing temples. He is the God that comes to me when I am at my lowest. He comes to meet me in my feeble state to take me to Himself and make me whole. He is the God who cares for us when we are hurting. I see the hidden pain and anguish in those that I encounter daily. I share in the struggle at the hospital while they desperately look for answers but are really searching for God's loving touch. I believe that Jesus Christ, because of His love for us, shares in our suffering and pain as we are crucified with Him while in a hospital bed. He is there with us in that moment of darkness and during the horror of cancer and all the other terrible diseases even when we are not aware of His presence.

After all these experiences of pain and hurt, the only thing that really makes a difference is the knowledge that God is there with us. This revelation of God's presence happens when we recall and relive all the wonderful things God did for humanity and for all of us. The healing ministry at the hospital opened my heart to the graces God revealed to me in abundance through my history, my stories, and testimonies. They were once like the dusty pebbles that the young men found in the cave but that became stories of grace and healing once the light of God touched them ever so softly. These stories make us aware of God's presence and glory. Those little encounters with God speak volumes to us. They add relevance and make us aware of God's presence and unconditional love. God becomes real through each and every encounter and through each and every moment that becomes part of our story. Without His presence, those stories would be simple dusty pebbles devoid of value. However, God is present in each story and uses them to bestow His grace. These experiences of grace bring comfort when we are at our worst and lost.

Jesus says, "Come to me all you who are weary and burdened, and I will give you rest" (Matthew 11:28).

While visiting patients these days, I stand in awe and humble respect by their bedside. I have the privilege of witnessing the crosses they share with Christ as they lie in bed. I allow myself to be broken with those I encounter. I can comfortably say that I enjoy being at the hospital only by God's grace. I cannot ask God for a better ministry than serving Him while serving others at the most vulnerable times of their lives. I am with them in those sacred moments, and that is a privilege. I feel their pain, their fears, their struggles, and see their tears. I hear their questions, and I journey with them through the process until they find their answers. These patients allow me to partake in that vulnerability, and I enter that vulnerable space with love and respect.

I have come to realize that no answers seem like they are enough when we are suffering. No answer will make sense in that pit of despair. Instead of trying to come up with the perfect "catchphrase" or the most compassionate words, I see the power of grace ever so present when I sit in silence and listen to the sick. I show compassion for their physical and spiritual wounds. I know in my heart that our love for patients is rooted in compassion. The depth of our love of God, commitment to our faith and what we believe in, our love and devotion to care for patients make me proud to be part of the team. I pray that the trials and crosses we are carrying will be a means of experiencing the full blissfulness of God. The reality is that horror is indeed present when we have to endure pain and grieve losses, but the grace of God is also overwhelmingly present. I believe like Saint Paul that "the Lord who has started the good work in us will bring it to completion" (Philippians 1:6).

This passage of scripture mirrors my perception of my journey so far working in the ministry of healing and providing care at the hospital. Saint Paul says,

> I thank my God every time I remember you. In all my prayers for all of you, I always pray with joy because of your partnership in the gospel from the first day until now, being confident of this, that he who began a good work in you will see it to completion until the day of Christ Jesus. (Philippians 1:3)

It is there where I find the foundation for my love, respect and appreciation for those I meet along the journey. The fears I experienced at the beginning of what would become my ministry are no more as I know that God continues to fill the void of my inadequacies. I have seen His grace in the horror of pain, loneliness hopelessness, and despair, but it is the horror in the journey to grace that has taught me the most.

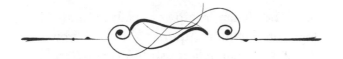

Reading List

These books and articles had great influence in my ministry and experiences at the hospital. However, some of them were not directly quoted in this book.

Alves, Rubem A. *The Poet, The Warrior, The Prophet*. London: SCM Press, 2002.

Alves, Rubem. *Transparencies of Eternity*. Miami, Florida: Continuum Press, 2010.

Butler, Sarah A. *Caring Ministry, A Contemplative Approach to Pastoral Care*. New York: Continuum, 2005.

Carretto, Carlo. *Why O Lord? The Inner Meaning of Suffering*. New York: Orbis Books, 1986.

Endo, Shusaku. *Silence*. New York: Picador, 2016.

Evans, Abigail Rian. *Is God Still at the Bedside? The Medical, Ethical, and Pastoral Issues of Death and Dying*. Grand Rapids, Michigan: William B. Eerdmans Publishing Company, 2011.

Frankl, Viktor. *Man's Search for Meaning*. Boston, Mass.: Beacon Press, 2006.

Friedman, Edwin H. *Generation to Generation: Family Process in Church and Synagogue*. New York: Guilford, 1985.

Frost, Ron. "The Relationship of Nature and Grace in the Theology of Thomas Aquinas." https://growrag.wordpress.com/2014/05/18/the-relationship-of-nature-and-grace-in-the-theology-of-thomas-aquinas-juxtaposed-with-augustine/.

Fujimura, Makoto. *Silence and Beauty*. Illinois: IVP Books, 2016.

Hiltner, Seward. *Pastoral Counseling*. New York: Abingdon Press: 1949.

Kushner, Harold S. *When Bad Things Happen to Good People*. New York: Anchor Books, 2004.

Most Bible quotations are from The Study Bible, New International Version, Michigan: Zondervan, 2016. and http://www.usccb.org/bible

Nicodemus Tebatso Makhalemele. "The Theology of Sickness and Suffering According to John Paul II: A Contribution Towards Pastoral Care of the Sick." https://ost.edu/theology-sickness-suffering-according-john-paul-ii-contribution-towards-pastoral-care-sick/.

Nolan, Simon F. "The Philosopher Pope: Pope John Paul II & the Human Person." http://www.carmelites.ie/PhilosopherPope.pdf.

Olson, Roger. "The Dialectic of 'Nature and Grace' in Christian Theology." https://www.patheos.com/blogs/rogereolson/2015/04/the-dialectic-of-nature-and-grace-in-christian-theology/.

Paul II, John. "On the Christian Meaning of Human Suffering." http://www.vatican.va/content/john-paul-ii/en/apost_letters/1984/documents/hf_jp-ii_apl_11021984_salvifici-doloris.html.

Schroeder, Robert G. *John Paul II and the Meaning of Suffering: Lessons from a Spiritual Master*. Indiana: Our Sunday Publishing, 2008.

Soelle, Dorothee. *Suffering*. Philadelphia: Fortress Press, 1975.

Saint Augustine, "On Grace and Free Will." http://www.newadvent.org/fathers/1510.htm.

Steinke, Peter L. *Congregational Leadership in Anxious Times,* Virginia: The Alban Institute, 2006.

Taylor, Kylea. *The Ethics of Caring: Honoring the Web of Life in Our Professional Healing Relationships*. California: Hanford Mead, 1995.

Tolstoy, Leo *The Death of Ivan Ilyich,* Translated by Lynn Solotaroff, New York: Bantam Classic 2004.

West, Christopher. *Theology of the Body Explained: A Commentary of John Paul II's Man and Woman He Created Them*. Boston: Pauline Books and Media, 2007.

West, Christopher. *At the Heart of the Gospel: Reclaiming the Body for the New Evangelization*. New York: Image Books, 2012.

Wicks, Robert J. *Night Call: Embracing Compassion and Hope in a Troubled World*. New York: Oxford University Press, 2018.

Wicks, Robert J. *Bounce: Living the Resilient Life*. New York: Oxford University Press, 2010.

Catechism of the Catholic Church, New York: Image, 1997.
https://en.wikipedia.org/wiki/It_Is_Well_with_My_Soul
https://en.wikipedia.org/wiki/Gratia_non_tollit_naturam,_sed_perficit
https://in.pinterest.com/pin/758926974684892771/

About the Author

Modestus Ngwu, O.P. is a Dominican priest. He was born in Nigeria and has been a priest for more than fifteen years. He was ordained a priest in Nigeria before being sent to Saskatoon, Canada, where he worked for seven years in different ministries both as a pastor and a chaplain in the High Schools and prison. After his ministry there, he was assigned to USA in the diocese of Harrisburg, Pennsylvania, and works at the Hershey Medical Center, Pennsylvania, as a chaplain. He completed his Clinical Pastoral Education Residency Program at this same hospital. Currently he lives at St. Joan of Arc parish in Hershey where he also ministers.